Archetype, Attachment, Analysis

Archetype, Attachment, Analysis is a well-researched and thoroughly documented presentation of new material that offers a revision and reinterpretation of Jung's archetypal hypothesis, and examines the emergence of symbolic meaning in the human mind, both in early development and as a crucial feature of the analytic process.

With few exceptions, psychoanalysts since Freud have repudiated the significance of neurobiology, and have largely ignored psychology. Through ground breaking exploration of expanding knowledge and research evidence from other disciplines such as cognitive science, developmental psychology, and attachment theory, Jean Knox sheds important new light on Jungian theory and practice. Using information gathered through laboratory investigations and natural observational studies Jean Knox brings the notion of archetypes up to date and considers the implications of new paradigms for clinical work with patients.

Archetype, Attachment, Analysis is essential reading for all professionals and students of analytical psychology, and of great interest to psychotherapists, attachment theorists and psychologists.

Jean Knox is a psychiatrist and a professional member of the Society of Analytical Psychology, in private practice as a Jungian analyst. She is editor of the *Journal of Analytical Psychology* and a member of the Executive Committee of the International Attachment Network.

Archetype, Attachment, Analysis

Jungian psychology and the emergent mind

Jean Knox

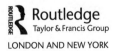

Routledge
Taylor & Francis Group

LONDON AND NEW YORK

First published 2003 by Brunner-Routledge
This edition published 2012 by Routledge
27 Church Road, Hove, East Sussex, BN3 2FA

Simultaneously published in the USA and Canada by Routledge
711 Third Avenue, New York NY 10017

Routledge is an imprint of the Taylor & Francis Group, an informa business

Typeset in Times by Mayhew Typesetting, Rhayader, Powys

Paperback cover illustration by Anthony Whishaw
Paperback cover design by Anú Design

British Library Cataloguing in Publication Data
A catalogue record for this book is available from the British Library

Library of Congress Cataloging-in-Publication Data

Knox, Jean, 1948-
    Archetype, attachment, analysis : Jungian psychology and the emergent
mind / Jean Knox.
        p. cm.
Includes bibliographical references.
    ISBN 1-58391-128-6 (alk. paper) – ISBN 1-58391-129-4 (pbk. : alk.
paper)
1. Archetype (Psychology) 2. Attachment behavior. 3. Jungian
psychology. I. Title.

    BF175.5.A72K68 2003
    150.19'54–dc21

                                                    2003005123

ISBN 978-1-58391-128-0 (hbk)
ISBN 978-1-58391-129-7 (pbk)

Contents

Acknowledgements

This book is about the emergence of symbolic meaning in the human mind, both in early development and as a crucial feature of the analytic process. I hope that it will therefore be of interest not only to analytical psychologists but also to psychotherapists, attachment theorists and psychologists whose professional trainings cover a wide theoretical spectrum and who want to discover more about a developmental approach to the emergence of subjective meaning in the mind.

Two main theoretical and clinical strands are interwoven throughout the book – analytical psychology and attachment theory – and I have greatly benefited from the encouragement and advice of experts who themselves come from many different fields.

The three people to whom I owe the greatest debt of gratitude are Peter Fonagy, John Morton and the late Anthony Storr. Anthony's initial help and encouragement were invaluable, but he died when the book was still in progress. I think he would have liked the finished product. John and Peter have done nothing less than revolutionize my approach to the human psyche, when they were my joint PhD supervisors. They taught me how to undertake conceptual research and to explore the similarities and differences in models of the mind derived from their respective disciplines. I hope that this book is a worthy reflection of the high standards they set.

I am also extremely grateful to my colleagues and friends who have given me helpful comments on various parts of the book. In particular, Joe Cambray and Margaret Wilkinson have been unfailingly generous with their advice and suggestions. I am also grateful to Ann Casement, Sue Gerhardt, Paul Gilbert, George Hogenson, Annette Karmiloff-Smith, Christopher Perry and David

Rosen for their comments and advice. I would also like to thank those people whose case material is included in this book with their permission. Pramila Bennett has provided invaluable help in preparing and checking the text. I am also grateful to Kate Hawes of Taylor & Francis for her encouragement and advice. Finally, my thanks go especially to my husband John and daughter Olivia, who have supported me throughout this work.

Jean Knox

Foreword

Freudian psychoanalysis and the natural sciences

Peter Fonagy

Historically, both Freudian and Jungian psychoanalysts have attempted to define their field independently of two major branches of scientific activity which pertain to their field: neurobiology and psychology.

With notable exceptions, psychoanalysts since Freud have repudiated the relevance of *neurobiology* to psychoanalytic ideas. The pressures of caring for patients and the inadequacy of neuroscience combined to make psychoanalytic science primarily a form of psychology, ultimately concerned only with ensuring that psychological treatment was provided in the most systematic and disciplined manner possible. The rejection of biology was not arbitrary but reasoned – not political but conceptual. There were clearly many reasons including the following: first, psychoanalysts were powerfully influenced by Freud's failure to create a psychoanalytic neurobiology (Freud 1895) and opted for a purely mentalistic model based around verbal reports of internal experience. Second, in the 1940s and 1950s neurobiology was dominated by mass action theory (Lashley 1923, 1929) which held that the cortex was largely indivisible from a functional point of view and behaviour could not be usefully studied from the point of view of the brain. Third, neuroscientists were, by and large, unconcerned with mental health problems, their focus being on deficits of cognitive functioning rather than affect regulation. Fourth, psychoanalysis evolved in radical opposition to a prevailing view that mental disorders represented a constitutional vulnerability of the individual, which could not be remedied by environmental manipulations. Fifth, an unhelpful distinction between so-called functional and so-called organic disorder was accepted within psychiatry and other mental health professions, which although rarely scrutinized from this point of view, ultimately implied the acceptance of a mind–body dualism.

While in general, in terms of the quality of patient care and the development of the discipline of psychoanalysis, particularly the unwavering focus on unconscious determinants, it may have been helpful to isolate psychoanalysis from the brain sciences, a number of by-products of this isolationist stance have created problems as the original objections to a closer link between the two disciplines began to shift. Since the early 1970s there has been a revolutionary advance in all the neurosciences, which negated all the historical reasons for the isolated development of psychoanalysis (Solms and Turnbull 2002; Westen 1998; Westen and Gabbard 2002a, 2002b). If Freud were alive today he would have an enormously complex set of findings and theories to draw upon in reconceptualizing his 'Project for a scientific psychology' (Freud 1895) and would be hardly likely to abandon the enterprise of developing a neural model of behaviour. Much is now known about the way the brain functions, including the development of neural nets, the location of specific capacities with functional positron emission tomography and neuroscientists can hardly be said to be exclusively concerned with cognitive disabilities or so-called organic disorders (Kandel 1998; LeDoux 1995, 1997).

Genetics has progressed, if anything, even more rapidly and mechanisms which underpin and sustain a complex gene–environment interaction belie original naïve assumptions about constitutional disabilities (Plomin et al. 1997). To take just a small sample of significant leaps forward which such scientific progress generates in the delivery of mental health care: the effectiveness of selective serotonin re-uptake inhibitors (SSRIs) in both depression and obsessive-compulsive disorder (Joffe et al. 1996; Piccinelli et al. 1995), the undoubted benefits for children suffering from attention deficit hyperactivity disorder to be treated with methylphenidate (Fonagy 1997; Fonagy et al. 2002), the relative efficacy of neuroleptics in psychosis (Barbui and Saraceno 1996; Barbui et al. 1996), the growing recognition concerning the lack of efficacy of prolonged periods of hospital care and – its counterpart – the benefits of assertive community treatment (Holloway et al. 1995; Johnstone and Zolese 1998), the potential for early diagnosis via brain imaging of neurosurgically treatable lesions (Videbech 1997) etc. In fact, since the early 1980s the field of neuroscience has been wide open for input from those with an adequate understanding of environmental determinants of development and adaptation.

Paradoxically, the response of psychoanalysts has been generally defensive rather than welcoming of these remarkable advances in knowledge. Notwithstanding the commitment of most individual analysts to embracing all understanding, however painful and anxiety provoking, by and large the response of the psychoanalytic community has been unnecessarily dismissive and critical of many of these developments. The response has been as to an encroachment, withdrawing further and further into increasingly specialist areas rather than seeking to join and develop together with the evolution of brain science. The irrational prevailing belief appears to be that hard-won psychoanalytic insights could somehow 'be destroyed' rather than elaborated and enriched by the new methods of inquiry.

A further obstacle generated by the dichotomization of biology and patient care has been the anti-intellectual tendency of many psychoanalytic groups (Kandel 1998). There is an assumed incompatibility between an astute and acute attention to the mental state of the patient. It is as if our observation of intellectualization in our patients could somehow be automatically generalized to our own activities: from observing that a patient who reads and talks about science rather than feelings is not doing analysis, we appear to assume that an analyst who reads science also cannot be feeling and therefore cannot be practising analysis. There is an obvious element of truth in this attitude in so far as reading and keeping up with science is time consuming and must take away from time devoted to clinical work. However, to claim that the two activities are hostile to one another is clearly an expression of prejudice rather than fact and somewhat self-serving on the part of those who do not wish to engage in such activities. Fortunately, the generation of psychoanalytic clinicians whose original professional training has already encompassed the rapid advances we are discussing neither understands, nor can have much sympathy with, this approach.

The psychoanalytic *attitude to psychology* mirrors the attitude of psychoanalytic psychiatrists to experimental medicine and the rest of biology. Progress in psychology has been largely ignored by psychoanalysts, despite the fact that an increasing number of psychoanalytic practitioners received their basic training in clinical psychology. Again, historically there are a number of valid reasons for this: first, psychology until the 1960s had an almost exclusive concern with behaviour and its models were largely based on studies of learning in animals (Skinner 1953). Second, psychology traditionally had an antagonistic attitude to psychoanalysis, seeing it as a major, medically dominated rival in offering psychological care in mental health settings (Eysenck 1952). Third, psychology retained a positivist influence upon its epistemology longer than most other social science disciplines. In fact its liberation from positivism is as much to be credited to progress in disciplines such as linguistics and sociology as to progress within its own domains (Chomsky 1968). Fourth, principally as a consequence of the previous factors, clinical psychology was frequently purposely naïve in its approach to the evaluation and treatment of mental disorder (Ullmann and Krasner 1969; Wolpe 1969) – a naivety that was abhorrent to psychoanalysts who had fought hard to acquire a sophistication concerning the nature of mental processes and mental phenomena.

About the same time as the revolution began in the brain sciences, psychology underwent a radical transformation, moving it from the periphery of the study of the mind to its current position as the recognised leader in the scientific study of mental processes (Westen 1999). The chief driving forces behind these changes were, first, the elaboration of the computer metaphor for psychological processes and the use of computer modelling for testing the appropriateness of psychological theories (e.g. Schmajuk et al. 1998). Second, the harnessing of technology for improved quality of observation, including the ready availability of video recordings, improved physiological measurements, endocrine and genetic analysis (e.g. Plomin et al. 1997). Third, more sophisticated methods of data analysis including techniques for causal analysis and special methods for analysing large data sets (McClelland 1997). Fourth, recognizing the limitations of their early attempts at psychological intervention, clinical psychologists have worked hard to provide adequate psychological treatments, rarely seeing themselves in opposition to other treatment approaches, but rather as adjuncts bridging the gaps which cheaper pharmacological treatments left behind (Salzman 1998; Thase 1997). Fifth, by contrast to the attitude of psychoanalysts, psychologists embraced and built upon developments in related fields and have undertaken many significant large-scale collaborative investigations (e.g. Offord et al. 1992; Rutter et al. 1981).

The problems created by the combination of psychoanalytic prejudice against non-medical disciplines in general and psychology in particular have grown over the years. One aspect of the problem is the voluntary abandonment by psychoanalysis of opportunities for major contributions to the behavioural sciences. A good instance of this is the controversy concerning developmental studies (Green 2000; Wolff 1996). The attempt to reduce psychoanalytic developmental work to a mere metaphor flies in the face of Freud's intentions as indicated by his own observational studies (see Freud 1909, 1919, 1920) as well as the work of some of the most distinguished psychoanalytic clinicians including Anna Freud, René Spitz, Margaret Mahler, Esther Bick, Donald Winnicott – all of whom saw value in observing the young child, particularly in interaction with a caregiver. These efforts have been meaningful sources of inspiration to theory building and to draw a sharp line between observational studies and psychoanalytic theory as a matter of principle at this particular time seems arbitrary, unscientific and counter-productive. There is no discernible rationale except apparent incompatibilities between the psychoanalytic theories arising out of psychoanalytic observation and those cherished by certain theoreticians. To suddenly rule out observations because these no longer fit in with preconception is certainly not what Freud taught us about science. The scientific developmental model has never been metaphorical – nor has it ever been closer to empirical validation (see, for example, Westen 1998). For example, while Anna Freud and Glover criticized Klein for the extravagant developmental claims implied by her theory, more recent observational evidence is by and large consistent with her claims – certainly those in terms of the cognitive capacities of the human infant (Gergely 1991).

There is an even more problematic area concerning psychological therapies where the isolationist attitude of psychoanalysts has undoubtedly created a long-term problem. The pressure for cheaper, more cost-effective therapies has prompted some psychoanalytic clinicians to experiment with alternative methods of treatment – briefer, more focused therapies, special therapies for particular groups (e.g. Malan and Osimo 1992; Sifneos 1992). These experiments were, on the whole, poorly supported by the psychoanalytic establishment, which might have been over-concerned about the apparent superficiality of brief therapy. The gap was rapidly filled by alternative therapies, with often very limited observational or theoretical basis, borrowing increasingly heavily, and relatively openly, from psychoanalytic discoveries (e.g. Ryle 1994). This has reached a point where certain schema focused therapies which represent an extension of the cognitive behavioural tradition are hard to differentiate from psychoanalytic therapies (Meichenbaum 1997; Young 1990). We have tried to show that psychoanalytic technique is only illusorily based on psychoanalytic theory. Both the discoveries and the effects of cognitive behavioural therapy and even behaviour therapy, are as easy to explain in terms of psychoanalytic ideas as in terms of behavioural ones (Fonagy 1989; Wachtel 1977). It seems, therefore, regrettable that psychoanalysts have not been more vigorous since the late 1970s in experimenting with and evolving new psychotherapeutic techniques, but rather rigidly sticking to the 'one size fits all' principle. They abandoned the field of technical innovation to psychologists who, in part at least because of the opposition of psychoanalysts, have come to define themselves as 'new and innovative' in contrast to psychoanalytic ideas.

This situation has altered somewhat, but only over very recent years. Many US institutes of psychoanalysis have started training psychotherapy candidates, only some of whom are expected to go on to full psychoanalytic training. Others have accepted directly the challenge of alternative therapies and are either working towards integrating effective components of these into psychoanalytically oriented treatments (Goldfried 1995) or are working towards differentiating the effective elements of each (e.g. Jones 1997). There is still a major gap in the integration of psychoanalysis and psychology, particularly in taking on board the major advances that the controlled, experimental study of human mental processes has brought to the psychology of language, perception, memory, motivation, emotion, development, social relationship and so on.

The geneticist Eric R. Kandel (1998) argued in a convincing way that

> the future of psychoanalysis, if it is to have a future, is in the context of an empirical psychology, abetted by imaging techniques, neuro-anatomical methods, and human genetics. Embedded in the sciences of human cognition, the ideas of psychoanalysis can be tested, and it is here that these ideas can have their greatest impact.
>
> (Kandel 1998: 468)

Jungian psychoanalysis and the natural sciences

In many ways Freud and Jung parted company over the issue of dynamic psychology's relation to natural science. Freud, as we know, embraced the respectability which natural science offered. Jung's epistemology, while not directly hostile to nineteenth-century versions of scientific thought, was clearly inconsistent with the positivist epistemology of twentieth-century science. Freudian psychoanalysis struggled with its natural science heritage throughout the century, with analysts periodically attempting to integrate or at least accommodate to epistemologies quite hostile to psychoanalytic thinking in order to regain the Freudian ideal of psychoanalysis as the science of the mind. As we know, throughout most of the twentieth century, this was not either a particularly successful nor a particularly popular line of thinking. Scientific giants such as George S. Klein, Merton Gill and their inspiration, David Rapaport, as well as journals such as *Psychoanalysis and Contemporary Thought*, represent some of the high-water marks of these initiatives.

In the mean time, Jungian psychoanalysis felt it could afford to ignore developments in scientific thought. Many in the Jungian academic community chose to highlight the more romantic/mystical aspects of Jung's writings, and others who moved closer to Freudian psychoanalysis chose object relations ideas in preference to ego-psychological ones. Thus, Jungian analytical psychology remained at some distance from the scientific revolution that took place in the last decades of the twentieth century.

Jean Knox's book is the first serious attempt to integrate aspects of Jungian psychoanalysis with the explosion of knowledge in neuroscience and psychology. The book centres around the concept of archetypes, a central idea in Jungian psychology. It uses information gathered through laboratory investigations and natural observational studies to bring the notion of archetypes up to date. It is the aptness of many of Jung's ideas in the context of new research findings which is so striking about this book. Also important is the even-handedness with which Jean Knox evaluates evidence which has emerged. There is no hint of selective use of information to prove cherished points; rather, the entire breadth of developmental and cognitive science research is taken on board to be scrutinized from the point of view of its value in elaborating the concept of archetypes. This exercise in itself is enormously valuable to those working within a Jungian model. They can obtain a completely fresh and creative perspective on 'old' ideas which suddenly become different, exciting and new, charged with the perspective of brain development and new knowledge on the way attachment relationships evolve to organize the social and mental world. But the book goes beyond this and exposes the theoretical insights to the challenge of clinical explanation. The second half of the book is principally concerned with clinical phenomena and the way in which ideas from developmental science can enlighten us in our understanding of clinical conditions. The review includes a stunning synthesis of the implications of developmental theory for our understanding of therapeutic change.

Throughout the book an understanding of archetypes emerges as a non-mystical but profound representation of the deep organizing unconscious, which cognitive science has finally helped us understand as a mechanism. To understand lasting change as occurring within this system sets us both a theoretical and clinical challenge. Bringing the developmental perspective to the notion of archetypes and Jungian psychology in general is the major contribution of this volume. It is, however, also significant as the first of perhaps many similar studies that will bring the excitement of Jungian ideas together with the powerful new knowledge from neuroscience. This is a pioneering and revolutionary book that will open the eyes of many with a Jungian training to an exciting new world. I think it will also serve a function in helping those who have rejected Jung's ideas on the basis of what turns out to be epistemological prejudice to see merit and value in the work of the second great originator of psychoanalytic thought. The connection between Freud and Jung has strengthened over the decades. This book is a further milestone in this process of rapprochement.

References

Barbui, C. and Saraceno, B. (1996) 'Low-dose neuroleptic therapy and extrapyramidal side effects in schizophrenia: an effect size analysis', *European Psychiatry*, 11: 412–15.

Barbui, C., Saraceno, B., Liberati, A. and Garattini, S. (1996) 'Low-dose neuroleptic therapy and relapse in schizophrenia: meta-analysis of randomized-controlled trials', *European Psychiatry*, 11: 306–13.

Chomsky, N. (1968) *Language and Mind*, New York: Harcourt, Brace.

Eysenck, H.J. (1952) 'The effects of psychotherapy: an evaluation', *Journal of Consulting Psychology*, 16: 319–24.

Fonagy, P. (1989) 'On the integration of psychoanalysis and cognitive behaviour therapy', *British Journal of Psychotherapy*, 5: 557–63.

—— (1997) 'Evaluating the effectiveness of interventions in child psychiatry: the state of the art – part II', *Canadian Child Psychiatry Review*, 6: 64–80.

Fonagy, P., Target, M., Cottrell, D., Phillips, J. and Kurtz, Z. (2002) *What Works for Whom? A Critical Review of Treatments for Children and Adolescents*, New York: Guilford.

Freud, S. (1895) 'Project for a scientific psychology', in J. Strachey (ed.) *The Standard Edition of the Complete Psychological Works of Sigmund Freud* (vol. 1, pp. 281–93), London: Hogarth Press.

—— (1909) 'Analysis of a phobia in a five-year-old boy', in J. Strachey (ed.) *The Standard Edition of the Complete Psychological Works of Sigmund Freud* (vol. 10, pp. 1–147), London: Hogarth Press.

—— (1919) '"A child is being beaten": a contribution to the study of the origin of sexual perversion', in J. Strachey (ed.) *The Standard Edition of the Complete Psychological Works of Sigmund Freud* (vol. 17, pp. 175–204), London: Hogarth Press.

—— (1920) 'Beyond the pleasure principle', in J. Strachey (ed.) *The Standard Edition of the Complete Psychological Works of Sigmund Freud* (vol. 18, pp. 1–64), London: Hogarth Press.

Gergely, G. (1991) 'Developmental reconstructions: infancy from the point of view of psychoanalysis and developmental psychology', *Psychoanalysis and Contemporary Thought*, 14, 3–55.

Goldfried, M.R. (1995) *From Cognitive-Behavior Therapy to Psychotherapy Integration*, New York: Springer.

Green, A. (2000) 'Science and science fiction in infant research', in J. Sandler, A-M. Sandler and R. Davies (eds) *Clinical and Observational Psychoanalytic Research: Roots of a Controversy*, London: Karnac.

Holloway, F., Oliver, N., Collins, E. and Carson, J. (1995) 'Case management: a critical review of the outcome literature', *European Psychiatry*, 10: 113–28.

Joffe, R., Sokolov, S. and Streiner, D. (1996) 'Antidepressant treatment of depression – a meta-analysis', *Canadian Journal of Psychiatry*, 41: 613–16.

Johnstone, P. and Zolese, G. (1998) 'Length of hospitalization for those with severe mental illness (Cochrane Review)', *Cochrane Library* (vol. 4), Oxford: Update Software.

Jones, E.E. (1997) 'Modes of therapeutic action', *International Journal of Psycho-Analysis*, 78: 1135–50.

Kandel, E.R. (1998) 'A new intellectual framework for psychiatry', *American Journal of Psychiatry*, 155: 457–69.

Lashley, K.S. (1923) 'The behaviouristic interpretation of consciousness', *Psychological Review*, 30: 237–72, 329–53.

—— (1929) *Brain Mechanisms and Intelligence: A Quantitative Study of Injuries to the Brain*, Chicago: University of Chicago Press.

LeDoux, J. (1995) 'Emotion: clues from the brain', *Annual Review of Psychology*, 46: 209–35.

—— (1997) 'Emotion, memory and pain', *Pain Forum*, 6: 36–7.

McClelland, G.H. (1997) 'Optimal design in psychological research', *Psychological Methods*, 2: 3–19.

Malan, D. and Osimo, F. (1992) *Psychodynamics, Training and Outcome in Brief Psychotherapy*, London: Butterworth-Heinemann.

Meichenbaum, D. (1997) 'The evolution of a cognitive-behavior therapist', in J.K. Zeig (ed.) *The Evolution of Psychotherapy: The Third Conference*, New York: Brunner/Mazel.

Offord, D.R., Boyle, M.H., Racine, Y.A., Fleming, J.E., Cadman, D.T., Blum, H.M. *et al.* (1992) 'Outcome, prognosis and risk in a longitudinal follow-up study', *Journal of the American Academy of Child and Adolescent Psychiatry*, 31: 916–23.

Piccinelli, M., Pini, S., Bellatuno, C. and Wilkinson, G. (1995) 'Efficacy of drug treatment in obsessive-compulsive disorder: a meta-analytic review', *British Journal of Psychiatry*, 166: 424–43.

Plomin, R., DeFries, J.C., McLearn, G.E. and Rutter, R. (1997) *Behavioral Genetics*, 3rd edn, New York: W.H. Freeman.

Rutter, M., Tizard, J. and Whitmore, K. (eds) (1981) *Education, Health and Behaviour*, rev. edn, New York: Krieger.

Ryle, A. (1994) 'Psychoanalysis and cognitive analytic therapy', *British Journal of Psychotherapy*, 10: 402–5.

Salzman, C. (1998) 'Integrating pharmacotherapy and psychotherapy in the treatment of a bipolar patient', *American Journal of Psychiatry*, 155: 686–8.

Schmajuk, N.A., Lamoureux, J.A. and Holland, P.C. (1998) 'Occasion setting: a neural network approach', *Psychological Review*, 105: 3–32.

Sifneos, P.E. (1992) *Short-term Anxiety-provoking Psychotherapy*, New York: Basic Books.

Skinner, B.F. (1953) *Science and Human Behavior*, New York: Macmillan.

Solms, M. and Turnbull, O. (2002) *The Brain and the Inner World: An Introduction to the Neuroscience of Subjective Experience*, New York: Other Press.

Thase, M.E. (1997) 'Integrating psychotherapy and pharmacotherapy for treatment of major depressive disorder: current status and future considerations', *Journal of Psychotherapy Practice and Research*, 6: 300–6.

Ullmann, L.P. and Krasner, L. (1969) *A Psychological Approach to Abnormal Behavior*, Englewood Cliffs, NJ: Prentice-Hall.

Videbech, P. (1997) 'MRI findings in patients with affective disorder – a meta-analysis', *Acta Psychiatrica Scandinavica*, 96: 157–68.

Wachtel, P. (1977) *Psychoanalysis and Behaviour Therapy: Toward an Integration*, New York: Basic Books.

Westen, D. (1998) 'The scientific legacy of Sigmund Freud: toward a psychodynamically informed psychological science', *Psychological Bulletin*, 124(3): 333–71.

—— (1999) *Psychology: Mind, Brain, and Culture*, 2nd edn, New York: Wiley.

Westen, D. and Gabbard, G.O. (2002a) 'Developments in cognitive neuroscience: I. Conflict, compromise, and connectionism', *Journal of the American Psychoanalytic Association*, 50(1): 53–98.

—— (2002b) 'Developments in cognitive neuroscience: II. Implications for theories of transference', *Journal of the American Psychoanalytic Association*, 50(1): 99–134.

Wolff, P.H. (1996) 'The irrelevance of infant observations for psychoanalysis', *Journal of the American Psychoanalytic Association*, 44: 369–92.

Wolpe, J. (1969) *The Practice of Behavior Therapy*, New York: Pergamon.

Young, J.E. (1990) *Cognitive Therapy for Personality Disorders: A Schema-focused Approach*, Sarasota, FL: Professional Resource Exchange.

Chapter 1

Introduction

It is impossible to understand contemporary analytical psychology and psychoanalysis without knowing something of the fault lines that characterized the early days of depth psychology. In geology, tension builds where segments of the earth's crust are moving in different directions from each other, creating fault lines which give rise to sudden and violent seismic shifts. It is a metaphor which seems particularly appropriate to the world of depth psychology, which has experienced many such earthquakes in its history. The first of these occurred in 1913 when, after a period of increasing tension as Freud and Jung moved in different directions, they finally severed their relationship, creating a rupture between psychoanalysis and analytical psychology that persists to this day (Hayman 1999: 164). Furthermore, within each school, further fault lines have developed so that a multiplicity of theories, trainings and clinical practice sit uneasily alongside each other and occasionally give rise to further violent fractures. Within analytical psychology, these fault lines, marking major divisions in theory and practice, have been extensively mapped in Samuels' account of the main theoretical and clinical distinctions between the archetypal, classical and developmental schools and in Kirsch's history of the Jungians (Samuels 1985; Kirsch 2001).

The dilemma, which faces every practising analyst and psychotherapist, is that our clinical work requires both a highly developed hermeneutic understanding, a capacity to relate to and explore the subjective meaning of a patient's conscious and unconscious communications, and also a reasonable grasp of the current scientific evidence about the information-processing mechanisms that underpin subjective experience and meaning. The art of being an analyst requires us to attend to the intuitive, poetic, symbolic narrative that emerges in an analytic session. Peter Levi (1977) has described the way in which a good poet can help us to hear our language, just as an eighteenth-century sailor 'could pick out intuitively the sound of every strain or creak or squeak in a great ship at sea', a metaphor which could equally well describe the intuitive listening of a well-trained analyst or psychotherapist during a session (Levi 1977: 12). It is an art which requires years of personal analysis, training and supervision to nurture the capacity to resonate with the multiple and sometimes contradictory threads of the patient's narrative.

It also requires a deeply ingrained respect for the symbolic process. For example, analysts who enter into sexual relationships with their patients not only abuse the patient physically and misuse the power accorded to them by the patient's transference but also are engaging in a fundamental violation of the fragile co-construction of a symbolic space, a psychological abuse which may destroy the last hope that patient has of finding the symbolic 'holding' that is a prerequisite for individuation.

However, the art of sensitive responsiveness to a patient's subjective experience is necessary but not sufficient for clinical practice, because our interpretations are shaped, not only by the patient's material but also by the theoretical models that we draw on to understand that material. Unfortunately, both psychoanalysis and analytical psychology have insulated themselves for too long from the influence of empirical research in the evolving disciplines of developmental psychology, cognitive science, neuroscience and attachment theory. The result has been that the depth psychologies, while rich in hermeneutic understanding, are impoverished as empirical sciences and carry diminishing authority as scientific models for understanding the human psyche. There has been a huge gulf between depth psychology, with its focus on subjective experience, and academic psychology, rooted in experimental observation, which neither side has wanted to bridge until recently. Whittle (1999) has also used the metaphor of the fault line to describe this divide and suggests that some observers see it as an intellectual scandal. Until recently academic psychology has largely neglected the study of subjective experience and has therefore seemed sterile and irrelevant to many practising analysts and therapists. Psychodynamic models have therefore become increasingly out of touch with the wealth of recent experimental evidence which provides new insights into the ways in which the human mind registers, stores and accesses information about the world around us. Psychodynamic psychotherapists of all orientations were, until recently, mainly content to remain largely ignorant of the huge strides made by cognitive scientists in understanding the workings of the human mind. Many therapists to this day even seem proud of their ignorance of these other areas of study. They argue that the analytic session is itself a sufficient research tool and that therapists share their clinical experience and evidence with one another in seminars and in published clinical papers, believing that this provides accumulating knowledge about the human mind and the way it works.

However, Fonagy and Tallindini-Shallice (1993) have challenged this argument, pointing out the inherent bias of this approach, in that analysts interpret what they find in the clinical session in the light of their pre-existing expectations, assumptions and theoretical orientation. This 'enumerative inductivism', the finding of ever more examples consistent with the model being used, is essentially flawed in that its subjectivity means that it is an approach which is not capable of eliminating false positive observations; psychotherapists and analysts who rely on this method for their understanding of the human psyche have no means of modifying or discarding their theories once they have been accepted as plausible.

The absence of any objective criteria for testing psychodynamic models also provides an epistemological breeding ground in which multiple and competing theories about the development and functioning of the human psyche can emerge, as analysts construct new models to understand the clinical phenomena they encounter in the consulting room. The problem which then arises is that, as theories multiply, it becomes less and less possible for analysts to agree among themselves about the nature of the events taking place in an analytic session; the bias produced by the analyst's expectations reaches a point where no objective observation of fact is possible. For example, one American research project asked analysts to rate a transcript of an analytic session to see whether, in their view, an analytic process had been established. The alarming outcome of this study was that the raters, all experienced analysts, could not complete the task because they could not even agree on the criteria for evaluating whether an analytic process was taking place in the session (Vaughan *et al.* 1997).

This diversity of theoretical models may be acceptable from a post-modern perspective but it may be the source of considerable problems in the clinical situation. The intensely interpersonal nature of psychoanalytic work and the profound emotional dependence upon the analyst which the analysand develops results in a great vulnerability during the analysis for the analysand's sense of self, a vulnerability which is so much greater for those analysands whose sense of psychological self is already fragile. Fonagy proposed that patients who do not have an awareness of themselves as having minds rely on the therapist's reflective capacity to support and maintain their identities (Fonagy 1991); my own view is that this places a great responsibility on an analyst to offer to the patient a model of his or her psyche which is in keeping with the available evidence from cognitive science about the information-processing capacities of the human mind. I suggest, for example, that an analyst whose interpretations of the patient's communications always arise from an instinctual drive model deprives the patient of an opportunity to gain a deep understanding of the way in which past trauma may have been 'internalized' and so contributed to the patient's representational world.

Similarly, it is essential for analysts to understand that mental contents may be unavailable to conscious recall without repression being the mechanism involved. However repression is conceptualized, it always includes the idea that emotion plays a key role in keeping certain mental contents out of conscious awareness, but emotion may play no part at all in the fact that information stored in implicit memory is unavailable to consciousness. An analyst who insists that everything that is unavailable to consciousness must be emotionally repressed would be wrong theoretically; the clinical situation could also be confusing and persecutory to the patient if the analyst's interpretations imply that the patient's failure to remember is rooted in emotional resistance when the real reason is a failure of the retrieval process.

The dangers posed by a therapist of any theoretical orientation who has scientifically unsound models of mental functioning are most strikingly illustrated in relation to the controversial questions of false and recovered memory. Some therapists seem unaware of the complexity of memory processes, particularly the fact that memory is always a mixture of reconstruction and reproduction; they may put considerable pressure on their patients to 'recover' memories of past sexual abuse, without realizing that the constant focus on finding such material may lead the patient to imagine such events and perhaps eventually to come to believe that these imaginative representations are accurate representations of real past events. Other therapists may be unaware that memories can be forgotten for long periods of time and then recovered and may cause their patients distress if they fail to believe them.

These examples are given to illustrate my argument that therapists can mislead and confuse their patients in the clinical situation if they work with scientifically unsound models and theories about mental functioning. Just as we ask our patients to test and modify their distorted models of the world in analysis, so analysts must also be willing to subject ourselves to the same process. We fully understand this in terms of the need for personal analysis to reduce, as far as possible, the distortions of the patient's narrative by our own needs and anxieties. However, as a profession, we do not yet fully recognize that we also have to be open to intellectual influence, to the modifying and balancing evidence from other disciplines which can help to correct our theoretical distortions. The pioneers of depth psychology did recognize this and firmly embedded the hermeneutic aspect of clinical practice in theories about the workings of the human mind such as Freud's metapsychology, which was based on the state of scientific knowledge then available to him. Jung went further and undertook empirical testing of his theories early in his career, in the form of the word association test. However, these models have become frozen in the scientific framework of their day and have not been subject to the regular and frequent empirical testing which defines the scientific approach.

There is an urgent need for a reappraisal of many psychodynamic concepts in the light of the accumulating evidence from other disciplines and there seemed to be a turning point with the publication of Daniel Stern's (1985) *The Interpersonal World of the Infant*, which opened the eyes of much of the analytic community to the rich nourishment we could obtain from this kind of developmental research. Since then, both psychoanalysis and analytical psychology have begun to engage in this process, sometimes painful, of examining our theoretical models in the light of the rapid growth in scientific understanding of the workings of the human mind and brain. In this book, my aim is to contribute to this process by drawing on some of these recent discoveries to examine key areas of Jungian theory and practice. I will make particular use of research in attachment theory, which has already played a major part in the emergence of contemporary psychoanalytic models, but which, until recently, has not been used to explore key concepts in analytical psychology. Attachment theory is crucial to any examination of depth psychology because it combines the rigour of the scientific investigative method, while placing interpersonal relationships at the heart of its core concepts; it is a model which really does, for the first time, provide a bridge between the objectivity of academic and empirical psychology and the subjectivity of the hermeneutic approach (Grossman 1995). Attachment theory demonstrates that scientific understanding can be integrated with the narrative and interpersonal aspects of analytic work; the scientific and the hermeneutic do not need to be seen as contradictory, but instead the meaning-making process can itself become the object of scientific study.

Attachment theory developed out of the tensions over certain key issues in psychoanalysis, fault lines some of which were similar to those which had caused the rift between Freud and Jung so many years earlier. John Bowlby, the originator of attachment theory, was a psychoanalyst who became increasingly uneasy with the emphasis in psychoanalytic theory on autonomous intrapsychic processes, which seemed to him to be a solipsistic model which neglected the role of interpersonal relationships in the formation of the human internal world. He became particularly critical of the Kleinian model, which placed instinctual drive theory at the heart of psychoanalysis and which postulated that complex unconscious phantasy could arise in the earliest months of infancy as a direct expression of the libido or of the death instinct. Bowlby felt that this was a view which seemed to render the environment virtually insignificant in its contribution to the formation of psychic contents (Bowlby 1988: 43–4).

The argument over the degree to which innate processes and the environment respectively contribute to unconscious fantasy did not represent a new fault line in psychoanalysis. Ferenczi had already clashed with Freud over this issue and, in recognition of the impact of real experience and trauma on children, one of his papers was originally called 'The passions of adults and their influence on the sexual and character development of children' (Ferenczi 1933). The British Object Relations school, particularly Guntrip, Balint and Fairbairn, formed the definitive view that actual experience of the real world and of the key relationships in a child's life were internalized to form internal objects. This sharply contrasted with the Kleinian position, but British object relations theory as yet lacked some of the key features which Bowlby incorporated into an object relations model, so initiating the full flowering of attachment theory.

These additional features came from outside the world of psychoanalysis. Bowlby had become aware of the developing field of ethological research and he discovered the work of Lorenz, Tinbergen and Hinde. Out of his study of their work came his conviction that attachment is a 'primary motivational system', not rooted in hunger or instinctual drive, but an independent instinctual pattern of experience and behaviour. Striking support for his view came from the, by now, famous experiments by Harlow, who separated monkeys from their mothers at birth and then reared them with surrogate wire monkeys. Some of these 'mothers' had a feeding bottle attached to them and others had no bottle but were covered with a soft furry material. The infant monkeys clearly preferred the soft cloth 'mother', clinging to her for long periods and only turning to the wire monkey to feed (Harlow 1958). Once again, this kind of empirical research supported Bowlby's view of human psychological development as interpersonal, a view which has received support from developmental studies such as those of Stern and many others whose research has shown the inseparability of the intrapsychic and interpersonal.

An outline of this book

In analytical psychology, one of the main points of disagreement between different schools has centred on the nature of archetypes, their role in psychic functioning and their contribution to the process of change in analysis and therapy. In Chapter 2, I examine the complex and varied ways in which Jung wrote about archetypes. Many authors have commented on the conceptual confusion these writings convey and there would be nothing new in another book along these lines. In Chapter 2, I have therefore identified four fundamental conceptual descriptions of archetypes that regularly emerge in Jung's attempts to clarify and define them. Furthermore, the characteristics of each of these four models of archetypes can be defined by tracing their roots to one or other of a range of philosophical and scientific influences on Jung. This analysis of the four strands that are interwoven in the model of archetypes allows us then to examine how compatible they are with each other or whether, when combined, they create such an internally inconsistent definition of archetypes that it has to be modified to offer a more coherent model.

In addition, new light can be shed on the theoretical differences in analytical psychology and psychoanalysis if we bring the expanding knowledge from other psychological disciplines to bear on our differing approaches to the psyche. Indeed I will go so far as to suggest in this book that some, at least, of the apparently irreconcilable divisions between our theoretical frameworks can seem much less significant when viewed from a different perspective. In Chapter 3, I turn to the wealth of research that has emerged since the early 1990s in cognitive science and developmental psychology, which offer us new paradigms for understanding the relationship between genetic potential and environmental influence on the development of the human mind. The central theme here is that of self-organization of the human brain and the recognition that genes do not encode complex mental imagery and processes, but instead act as initial catalysts for developmental processes out of which early psychic structures reliably emerge. For example, the developmental account of archetype, which I offer in Chapter 3, lends considerable scientific support to the key role archetypes play in psychic functioning and as a crucial source of symbolic imagery, but at the same time identifies archetypes as emergent structures resulting from a developmental interaction between genes and environment that is unique for each person. Archetypes are not 'hard-wired' collections of universal imagery waiting to be released by the right environmental trigger, a model which would lead straight into the trap of categorizing them as innate ideas, a concept demolished by Locke long before anyone had ever heard of genes. Locke wrote:

> The knowledge of some truths, I confess is very early in the Mind; but in a way that shews them not to be innate. For, if we will observe, we shall find it still to be about ideas, not innate but acquired; it being about those first, which are imprinted by external things, with which infants have earliest to do, which make the most frequent Impressions on their senses.
>
> (Locke 1997 [1689]: 65)

This statement is breathtaking in its anticipation, more than 300 years ago, of a contemporary developmental understanding of the emergent nature of mental patterns.

The concept of mental models is fundamental to an information-processing approach to the human mind and this is the focus of Chapter 4. While image schemas can provide us with an information-processing model of the archetype-as-such, we also need to understand how day-to-day experience is internalized and structured into a pattern of core meanings. Research, much of it within an attachment theory framework, demonstrates that our expectations of the world are governed not by rules of formal logic but by implicit and explicit mental models which organize and give a pattern to our experience. The archetype, as image schema, provides an initial scaffolding for this process, but the content is provided by real experience, particularly that of intense relationships with parents and other key attachment figures stored in the form of internal working models in implicit memory.

Ainsworth's studies of secure and insecure attachment patterns in children have shown that the mother's responsiveness to her child is reflected in the child's pattern of attachment to her, as measured by the 'Strange Situation' (Ainsworth *et al.* 1978); Mary Main developed the Adult Attachment Interview (AAI), which showed that childhood patterns of attachment are internalized and stored in the internal working models which govern the attitudes and behaviour of a person in relationships (Main and Cassidy in press). Even more exciting is the fact that later studies have shown a correlation between parents' ratings on the AAI and the subsequent patterns of attachment of their children in the Strange Situation. It shows that it is not the parent's behaviour but his or her internal world which affects the child's pattern of attachment: the power of the unconscious in relationships is demonstrated for the most sceptical scientist to see.

In Chapter 5, I begin to examine some of the implications of these new paradigms for clinical work with patients by describing an attachment theory model of unconscious defences. Some people criticize attachment theory on the grounds that it is much too concerned with the real external world and not enough with the reality of unconscious fantasy that all analysts encounter in the consulting room. I shall show in Chapter 5 that attachment theory does in fact offer us a contemporary model in which unconscious fantasy is seen as truly psychological, as our way of protecting the self from unbearable reality and not as a secondary manifestation of a physiological phenomenon such as instinctual drive. Attachment theory places relationships at the centre of intrapsychic experience and so offers new ways of thinking about maladaptive and destructive patterns of relationship which therapists so often see in their patients; an important motivational factor in the perpetuation of attachment patterns is the desire to reproduce a familiar relationship pattern however destructive because it is familiar and understood. We all unconsciously seek out relationships with people who resonate with early attachment figures, however unsatisfactory they may have been.

A new area of research in attachment theory has been the nature of this unconscious communication from parent to child and its impact on the child's psychological development. The concept of reflective function has emerged to explain the vital role that the parent plays in facilitating the child's capacity to relate to other people as mental and emotional beings with their own thoughts, desires, intentions, beliefs and emotions. In Chapter 6 I trace the early manifestations of this capacity in the emergence of the 'theory of mind' at about the age of 3 years. I then analyse the nature of reflective function in more detail, showing that its full flowering depends on the ability to see that states of mind can be causal and on the capacity to make judgements, to have desires and appetites and to have a sense of one's own separate and unique identity. The full development of reflective function is probably the height of mental and emotional achievement, in that it reflects the full awareness of one's own and other people's humanity.

Chapter 7 examines the implications that the findings described in the previous chapters hold for our understanding of the process of change in analysis and therapy. Archetypes certainly play their part but in the form of image schemas which are experienced in non-verbal, implicit and embodied ways, rather than as pre-existing fully fledged symbolic meanings waiting to be activated. Instead, the activation of image schemas, or archetypes, in analysis may provide the first step towards the gradual emergence of the capacity to symbolize. The creation of narrative competence, the ability to connect past and present experiences together into a meaningful story is the next stage in this process. In addition, the uncovering of repressed meaning is not sufficient to bring about lasting change; new ways of relating to oneself and to others need to be slowly constructed in analysis, to emerge out of the transference and countertransference dynamics.

The main theme that runs through all the chapters of this book is that mind and meaning emerge out of developmental processes and the experience of interpersonal relationships rather than existing a priori. The emergence of archetypes out of the earliest stages of psychic development forms the foundation for the development of core meanings as we gradually construct mental models of the world around us, organizing day-to-day experience into patterns which can then guide our future expectations of life in all its aspects, including our expectations of relationships. At the highest levels of psychic complexity, the mature achievement of reflective function is also emergent and so is the creation of new patterns of meaning and relationship in analysis. At each level of complexity, the patterns that emerge are profoundly influenced by earlier stages of development but are also governed by their own constraints, the rules that operate at that particular level of complexity (Dupré 2001: 108). This is as true of the human mind as it is of the human body and at each stage of development the environment plays a key role in shaping the direction of each person's developmental potential. An account of this interaction, together with the forms that it takes, is the main purpose of this book.

Chapter 2

Jung's various models of archetypes

Both Freud and Jung were pioneers in the development of new models for understanding the human mind, models which they explored together until the traumatic rupture of their personal and professional relationship in 1913 (Hayman 1999: 163–4). One of the points on which they initially agreed was the idea that the human mind contained innate structures which play a large part in determining the way we perceive the world around us and which organize and give meaning to the multitude of information which our senses receive every second of our lives. This concept was revolutionary for its day, in that, in the first half of the nineteenth century, most psychologists thought the human mind was a *tabula rasa* with no innate content, structures or processes, and that it was entirely shaped by the environment. This behaviourist view also included the belief that 'the subjective inner states of mind, like perceptions, memories, and emotions, are not appropriate topics for psychology' (LeDoux 1998: 25). Stevens (2002) has coined the striking phrase 'psychic agnosticism' to describe this doubt that the psyche even exists, a position certainly adopted by one of the most famous behaviourists, B.F. Skinner, when he said that 'the question is not whether machines think but whether men do' (Pinker 1997: 62). Both these aspects of behaviourism became increasingly untenable in the mid-twentieth century, in the face of the information-processing approach of cognitive science and the exploration of possible innate mental processes by evolutionary psychologists (Dennett 1995; Fodor 1983; Pinker 1997; Barkow, Cosmides and Tooby 1992).

However, the question as to the nature of any innate mental structures has remained highly controversial from the start of the cognitive science revolution and is still largely unresolved. One of the pioneers of a developmental and conceptual model of the human mind, Jean Piaget, discarded the behaviourist paradigm, but did not consider that the mind has any innate content. Annette Karmiloff-Smith, who worked at the University of Geneva with Piaget, identifies similarities between some aspects of his constructivist model and behaviourism, while acknowledging that she risks the wrath of her former colleagues in doing so:

> Neither the Piagetian nor the behaviourist grants the infant any innate structures or domain-specific knowledge. Each grants only some domain-general, biologically specified processes: for the Piagetians, a set of sensory reflexes and three functional processes (assimilation, accommodation and equilibration); for the behaviourists, inherited physiological sensory systems and a complex set of laws of association. These domain-general learning processes are held to apply across all areas of linguistic and non-linguistic cognition. Piaget and the behaviourists thus concur on a number of conceptions about the initial state of the infant mind. The behaviourists saw the infant as a *tabula rasa* with no in-built knowledge (Skinner 1953); Piaget's view of the young infant as assailed by 'undifferentiated and chaotic' inputs is substantially the same.
>
> (Karmiloff-Smith 1992: 7)

Although academic psychology has changed enormously since the early 1950s, there is a considerable loss for psychology disciplines, such as those of evolutionary psychology and cognitive science, if they ignore the extent to which Freud and Jung anticipated some of their most exciting recent discoveries. The academic world of the early nineteenth century may be forgiven for its failure to grasp the full significance of concepts such as modularity (compartmentalization) and unconscious content in the human mind, concepts which are mapped out in a coherent way for the first time in Freudian and Jungian models of the human psyche. However, present-day academic psychologists are vulnerable to the kind of cogent criticism offered by one of their most eminent members, George Mandler, who wrote:

> Only the historical and theoretical ignorance of many cognitive psychologists prevents them from seeing that much of their work is consistent with, and often derives from, psychoanalytic concerns. Semantic networks, theories of forgetting, slips of

the tongue, the construction of consciousness, are all consistent with psychoanalytic theory.

(Mandler 1975: 3)

Some evolutionary psychologists do begin to integrate Freud's ideas into their own information-processing accounts of the human mind. Nesse and Lloyd (1992: 601), for example, suggest that some psychodynamic traits may turn out to closely match functional sub-units of the mind that are currently being sought by cognitive and evolutionary psychology. In their view the concepts used by psychoanalysts, such as those of repression, defences, intrapsychic conflict, childhood sexuality and transference, may not turn out to be the best categories for research but they are currently the best available as a description of processes occurring at this level of mental organization.

In contrast, the almost universal absence of any reference to Jung's model of the mind is puzzling, given the growing interest among cognitive scientists in some of the concepts such as dissociation and innate structures which Jung also explored. In the revised version of his book *Archetype Revisited* Anthony Stevens (2002) is equally critical of ethologists for their failure to acknowledge Jung's originality, writing:

> Nowadays, it is common to hear ethologists praised for their part in bringing psychology into the mainstream of biology; but those who deliver these accolades never give Jung his due for attempting a similar achievement, against almost universal opposition, so many years earlier.

(Stevens 2002: 29)

There are a few exceptions to this general neglect of Jung's work. Richard Lazarus, for example, has studied emotional appraisal for many years and acknowledges the value of Jung's work on symbolism and unconscious meaning (Lazarus 1991: 295). However, he does not link his own work with the concept of feeling function, which Jung used to refer to the evaluation of the meaning and significance of experience, an idea which seems very close to Lazarus's ideas of emotional appraisal. Other cognitive scientists have acknowledged the value of the word association test as a research tool but, on the whole, references to Jung are no more than passing comments (Kihlstrom and Hoyt 1990).

To analytical psychologists, it is particularly striking that the majority of academic psychologists who investigate innate mental processes make no mention of Jung's concept of the archetype. There are no references to Jung by Pinker (1994a, 1997), Dennett (1995) or Barkow, Cosmides and Tooby (1992), all of whose books explore the academic and research evidence for innate structures in the human mind. In the academic world, philosophers have shown the most interest and a few, notably Bishop, Brooke and Pietikainen, have contributed books and papers to the Jungian literature (Bishop 1999; Brooke 1991; Pietikainen 1998). One of the very few academic cognitive scientists to explore the links between Jung's concept of archetypes and the emerging ideas in evolutionary psychology about innate mental structures is Paul Gilbert. He attributes great importance to archetypes, describing them as 'the evolved psychological mechanisms of the mind which guide our behaviour in certain ways and have evolved (like the defence system) because they solved certain adaptive problems' (Gilbert 1995: 142).

Previous studies of the nature of archtypes

Most studies of the context for Jung's ideas have, to varying degrees, examined his theories within a particular frame of reference, perhaps in recognition of the fact that no researcher could ever be knowledgeable enough in all the areas which Jung studied to evaluate their relative significance in the evolution of his thinking. The problem arises from the multiplicity of influences which have been identified as contributing to Jung's emerging theories of archetypes. Ellenberger (1970) pointed out that:

> Much has been said about Jung's vast erudition. His early interests were in psychology and archaeology. Later, when he began to investigate the symbols, he acquired an extensive knowledge of the history of myths and religions. Among his particular interests were Gnosticism and alchemy, and later the philosophies of India, Tibet and China. Throughout his life he was greatly interested in ethnology. This variety of interests was reflected in his library.
>
> (Ellenberger 1970: 680)

A number of analysts and academics have undertaken the task of dissecting and clarifying the variety of ways in which Jung conceptualized archetypes, uncovering the main meanings which the ideas seemed to hold for Jung himself. One line of research has been to explore the range of philosophical, scientific, literary and religious sources which consciously or unconsciously influenced Jung's thinking and to show how his description of archetypes fluctuated as he explored the possibilities which each of these fields of knowledge offered him (Carrette 1994; Casement 2001).

Jolande Jacobi was one of the first Jungian theoreticians to identify the varied sources of the concept of archetype and to focus on the models which emerged from each of these sources. Her book *Complex/Archetype/Symbol* (1959) is a masterpiece of intellectual clarity, providing us with a valuable map of the influences on Jung's thinking, all of which she felt provided supporting evidence for archetypes, writing that 'The archetype can be approached from many angles. Jung has given us an almost inexhaustible store of statements on its diverse aspects' (Jacobi 1959: 35). Marie-Louise von Franz concurred with this view and also suggested that research into heredity would soon give us more exact information on the nature of archetypes, while valuing research into the relationship between archetypes and comparative religion and mythology (von Franz 1975: 126–7).

Ellenberger's monumental study *The Discovery of the Unconscious* (1970), mentioned already, included a chapter on Jung which was the most comprehensive analysis of his psychological system that had yet been written; he gives a summary of the key philosophers and psychiatrists, as well as theologians, mystics, orientalists, ethnologists, novelists and poets on whose works Jung had drawn. From this perspective, archetypes would be seen as the manifestations of the activity of a 'neo-Platonic world-soul'. Ellenberger tended to ignore the scientific heritage of which Jung considered himself an heir:

> Jung's analytical psychology, like Freud's psychoanalysis, is a late offshoot of Romanticism, but psychoanalysis is also the heir of positivism, scientism, and Darwinism, whereas analytical psychology rejects that heritage and returns to the unaltered sources of psychiatric Romanticism and philosophy of nature.
> (Ellenberger 1970: 657)

This statement fails to reflect Jung's sophisticated grasp of biology and of Darwinian concepts, most strikingly demonstrated when he wrote:

It is a mistake to suppose that the psyche of the newborn child is a *tabula rasa* in the sense that there is absolutely nothing in it. In so far as the child is born with a differentiated brain that is predetermined by heredity and therefore individualized, it meets sensory stimuli coming from outside, not with any aptitudes but with specific ones . . . These aptitudes can be shown to be inherited instincts and preformed patterns, the latter being the *a priori* and formal conditions of apperception that are based on instinct.

(Jung 1954[1936]: para. 136)

This statement is entirely in keeping with the most current biological research on the innate structures of the human mind and this aspect of Jung's concept of the archetype will be further investigated.

Ellenberger's work was followed in 1974 by *From Freud to Jung* by Liliane Frey-Rohn, who sidelines the scientific aspect of Jung's theory of archetypes to an even greater extent than Ellenberger. Although she does discuss the link between archetype and instinct, she makes the rather strange remark that this must never be mistaken for a biological assumption and says, incorrectly, that Jung never mentioned in his writings that psychic contents were in any way derived from the area of biology (Frey-Rohn 1974: 286). Her preference seems to be to see archetypes as rooted in the transcendental and non-psychic realm, a priori principles, or transpsychic ordering agencies. She draws on Jung's essay on synchronicity as evidence in support of her argument that archetypes derive from a transcendental reality, which he conceived as a kind of imperceptible space–time continuum.

Claire Douglas echoes Ellenberger and Frey-Rohn, emphasizing the Romantic influences on Jung's models of the mind rather than the scientific. She writes that 'Tracing the specific major sources of analytical psychology from the vast body of Jung's learning is a complicated task because it requires a knowledge of philosophy, psychology, history, art and religion' (Douglas 1997: 22). There is no mention of biology or the emerging discipline of ethology. Ann Casement's study of Jung also focuses more on the philosophical and religious, rather than the scientific, influences on his thinking, although she does highlight the important task of integrating Jung's ideas with recent neuroscientific research on the human mind and brain (Casement 2001: 133).

Roger Brooke (1991) has taken a phenomenological perspective on Jung's ideas, one which is also opposed to a scientific, biological analysis. Brooke interprets Jung's model of the psyche in the light of existential phenomenology; he argues that the natural-scientific theme in Jung's writing reflects a 'fatal defect' in his thinking because it maintains a false Cartesian subject–object split, in which subjective experience is considered to be less real than objective scientific evidence. Rauhala also takes the view that, although Jung used the language of early-twentieth-century psychology, 'the model of his thought is fundamentally that of phenomenology and philosophy of existence' (Rauhala 1984: 244)

A post-modern exploration of Jung's ideas by Christopher Hauke also rejects a classical scientific framework for the investigation of Jung's concept of archetypes. Although Hauke defines post-modernism as an approach that refuses to take 'truths' for granted and one in which claims for essentiality are questioned, he also suggests that archetypes represent a fundamental universal principle of acausal orderedness, akin to the *materia prima* of the alchemists (Hauke 2000: 257).

In striking contrast, Anthony Stevens (1982) has been, for some time, an acknowledged champion of Jung as a scientist, developing an evolutionary perspective on the concept of archetype. Stevens was the first since Jolande Jacobi to explore the archetype as a biological, instinctual entity, in *Archetype: A Natural History of the Self*. Stevens argues that

> there are indeed universal forms of instinctive and social behaviour, as well as universally recurring symbols and motifs, and that these forms have been subject to the essentially biological processes of evolution no less than the anatomical and physiological structures whose homologous nature first established the truth of Darwin's theory.
>
> (Stevens 1982: 47)

Stevens' subsequent publications have extended and developed this theme and his revised book *Archetype Revisited* unambiguously restates this position (Stevens 2002). A crucial feature of Stevens' position is his extension of the ethological perspective from 'patterns of behaviour' to 'pattern of awareness'. He points out:

> In contrast to Jung, ethologists are concerned with the outer manifestations of living organisms rather than with their

subjective experiences. For this reason, it would be a mistake to persist in a purely ethological orientation to the study of mankind because it would prevent a new scientific synthesis from occurring. There can be no unified science of humanity if it concentrates on the outer world of behaviour while ignoring the inner world of experience.

(Stevens 2002: 29)

Stevens argues with great passion that the failure of the ethological revolution to 'connect with the inside' can be redressed by Jungian psychology which forges this connection with the archetypal hypothesis.

Michael Fordham's developmental innovations in the theory and practice of analytical psychology are also based on his sound understanding of the importance of an evolutionary perspective on archetypes. In 'Biological theory and the concept of archetypes' (1957) he investigates the light which the emerging discoveries of ethology could shed on the characteristics of archetypes and came down firmly in favour of seeing them as biological entities:

It follows that when it is said that the archetypes are hereditary functions what is meant is that they must be somehow represented in the germ cells and that therefore any archetypal image recorded by the conscious mind likewise contains within it the effect of genetic factors.

(Fordham 1957: 11)

This effectively identifies the archetype-as-such with the genotype.

Anthony Storr also opts for the biological view of archetypes, rejecting the charge that Jung was Lamarckian and pointing out the similarity between the concept of archetypes and Tinbergen's innate release mechanisms (Storr 1973).

More recently, a steady stream of articles has begun to emerge by other authors who take up the scientific banner when investigating archetypes. Paul Gilbert is a rare example of a non-Jungian psychologist who understands the significance for academic psychology of the concept of archetypes as biological entities (1997: 35). An analytical psychologist and philosopher, George Hogensen (2001) has explored Jung's evolutionary thinking in the light of his knowledge of the work of neo-Darwinians such as Baldwin and Lloyd Morgan. Hogenson suggests that archetypes can be considered to be 'the emergent properties of the dynamic developmental system of brain, environment and narrative', rather than as pre-existing instructions hard-wired into the brain. This is also the view taken by Saunders and Skar (2001), although they extend this argument to conclude that archetypes should therefore be considered to be a special type of complex. However, this developmental model of the archetype is not entirely new and was spelt out as early as 1985 by Satinover, who wrote:

> Archetypal images need to be understood as the epigenetic consequence of developmental processes, certain elements of which (as may or may not be evident in the final product) are inherited. These heritable elements are the subject of ongoing research that has greatly altered traditional psychoanalytic theory in the direction of greater appreciation of what is innate (Campos *et al.* 1983). They ought to alter Jungian theory in the direction of greater appreciation of what is not innate.
>
> (Satinover 1985: 83)

Another perspective adopted by some authors is to view Jung's ideas in the light of his own psychology. One such work is a review of the psychological, religious and sociological influences on Jung's theories by Peter Homans (1979), who adopts a particular psychological viewpoint, that of Kohut's model of the psyche. This emphasis on understanding Jung's ideas as a particular form of narcissistic psychology leads Homans to argue that Jung dealt with his own intrapsychic conflicts by objectifying them. Homans argues that:

> This continuous process of objectification of alien feelings in the form of images, of engagement with these images, and of consequent interpretation of them made it necessary for him to formulate – to account for his own experiences – such concepts as the collective unconscious, the archetypes, differentiation of the ego from the contents of the collective unconscious through active imagination, the shadow, the anima, individuation, and the self.
>
> (Homans 1979: 83)

Homans suggests that, when writing *Symbols of Transformation* (1956), Jung had grandiosely and narcissistically fused the contents of his own consciousness with the mythological symbolism of the past, which then threatened to overwhelm him. He goes on to say:

> By constructing the theory of archetypes and all that goes with it, in one stroke – through the medium of thought itself – he interposed interpretative categories between his own mind and these cultural products, thereby separating himself from them.
> (Homans 1979: 83)

Homans' view of the concept of archetypes is, therefore, that they fulfilled a personally defensive role for Jung, and he investigates these psychological factors more extensively than cultural influences.

Renos Papadopoulos (1984: 63) also sees Jung's concept of the archetype as the culmination of his quest for a language and framework to describe the 'Other', and as an expression of his own personal search for meaning. Papadopoulos traces the connection between successive reformulations of the concept of the Other and the developmental stages of Jung's own life. He argues that Jung's sense of his 'Number Two personality' represents one early formulation of his struggle to identify the concept of the Other, a struggle which culminated in his formulation of the Other as Archetype.

Douglas (1997: 18) echoes Homans in arguing that the main themes in analytical psychology reflect Jung's own intrapsychic conflicts, but adopts a similar line to Papadopoulos in suggesting that they emerge out of the two opposing sides of Jung's own nature. One is the rational and enlightened side, which he called his Number One personality and which was demonstrated in his scientific empirical investigation of the psyche; the other side is the Romantic side drawn towards the unconscious, mysterious and hidden world of the psyche which he recognized as a reflection of his Number Two personality.

Several writers adopt a more neutral investigative stance. Andrew Samuels' (1985) *Jung and the Post-Jungians* is a valuable investigation of the main theoretical and clinical strands in contemporary analytical psychology, with one chapter examining the range of influences which contribute to the various meanings of the term 'archetype'. He acknowledges that Jung was profoundly influenced by both philosophy and biology, as well as by his experience as a psychiatrist (Samuels 1985). However, in his discussion of the archetype as blueprint, Samuels seems to concur with the view that accumulated human experience becomes stored as innate archetypal structures, a Lamarckian model which must be discarded in a post-Darwinian world and which Samuels himself modifies later in his book when he suggests that we should abandon the idea of discrete archetypes (Samuels 1985: 26–7).

Jung in Contexts also offers an overview of the range of intel-lectual disciplines which contributed to Jung's thinking, by means of a collection of essays, each of which explores a particular context for Jung's ideas (Bishop 1999). These focus mainly on a philosophical and literary perspective, with chapters on the influence of Hoffman, Nietzsche and Schopenhauer on Jung. However, these 'romantic' contexts are balanced by a rare exposition of the relationship between the central ideas of Jung's model of the psyche and those of the evolutionary orientated philosopher, Henri Bergson (Gunter 1999). In the same volume, John Haule investigates Jung's ideas in the context of the state of psychological understanding of their day. Haule suggests that Jung's concept of archetypes enable him to walk the tightrope between Freud's metapsychology, which focuses on latent Oedipal conflict as the source of all manifest psychological phenomena, and Janet's dissociationism, in which the focus is on the economics of the arousal and discharge of psychic energy rather than any specific content (Haule 1999: 260). The most recent biographer of Jung, Ronald Hayman (1999), has examined the development of Jung's models of the mind in the context of his personal history, while carefully avoiding any exploration of their relation to his personal psychological conflicts. He is another author who succeeds in giving a balanced picture of the range of influences on Jung's thinking and echoes Jolande Jacobi's view that it was not really considered important in Jung's day to distinguish between these influences, saying: 'Jung was lecturing over a hundred years ago, when science, philosophy and religion seemed to interpenetrate more than they do in the post-Einsteinian ethos' (Hayman 1999: 48).

One other author, Marilyn Nagy (1991), offers a rare integrated study of the philosophical and scientific influences contributing to Jung's concept of the archetype. She traces the original roots of this idea in Jung's differentiation of his concept of libido from that of Freud, explores the impact of biology on Jung's thinking and, finally, traces the influence of a number of philosophers, notably Plato, Kant and Schopenhauer, on his final formulations of the archetype. Nagy concludes:

The archetype itself, like the synchronistic event which reveals it, is 'the introspectively recognizable form of *a priori* orderedness'. Synchronistic events must be regarded as 'the continuous creation of a pattern that exists from all eternity . . . and is not derivable from any known antecedents'.

Such a formulation is very far from the biological 'pattern of behaviour'. It is far, too, from the theory of phylogenetic origins which Jung associated with his genetic theory of libido and then with his theory of archetypes. In spite of Jung's caveat against philosophical interpretation, it resembles nothing so much as Plato's vision of a universe ordered by the eternal forms, directed by the World Soul, and limited in the perpetration of divine order only by the parallel existing facts of Necessary Cause.

(Nagy 1991: 185)

Finally, one author, Carrette (1994: 185–6), conducts a review of the range of ideas that are interwoven in the concept of the archetype and comes to the conclusion that the confusion is so great that the applicability of the archetype is seriously questionable on the grounds of its phenomenological incoherence and that it 'has ceased to function effectively in relation to experience and phenomena, and has been magnified out of proportion to hold almost ontological value'.

This is not an exhaustive list of the writers who have examined the strands which have become interwoven in the concept of the archetype, but it does show the importance which many researchers have given to placing Jung's theories in a cultural and personal context, identifying the intellectual disciplines and the personal experiences from which those strands have been formed. Some of these studies adopt a neutral investigative approach, deliberately avoiding attributing greater significance to one context over others. Others, like Anthony Stevens and Roger Brooke, adopt the view that a more critical analysis of the concept of the archetype is required, and that this inevitably exposes inconsistencies between the contributing themes, some of which therefore have to be discarded. For Brooke, it is the scientific model which offers a false reading of the human psyche, while Stevens reckons that any view of the archetype which is not biologically sound must be abandoned.

The more we explore the intellectual influences that contributed to Jung's theories, the more we can see how impossible it is to argue that one particular view of archetypes is a more accurate reflection of Jung's views rather than another. However, we can examine the research which has been undertaken on the nature of archetypes to help us identify recurrent core ideas about the essential characteristics of what is generally accepted to be one of the most central concepts of Jungian theory. This approach reveals four main models, or concepts, which repeatedly emerge in each of the different disciplines within which the archetype has been explored. In subsequent chapters I hope to show how we can use contemporary cognitive and developmental research evidence to identify which of these concepts can rightly be labelled as innate and which play a role in other, non-innate aspects of human psychological functioning.

Core themes in Jung's concept of archetypes

One reason why Jung's ideas about innate mental structures have not penetrated the world of academic psychology may be the great complexity which many of the researchers I have mentioned have found in Jung's own writing about archetypes. This confusion arises out of the various meanings which the concept held for Jung himself at different times, under the influence of a range of ideological and conceptual frameworks which he drew on while he was struggling to develop his own theories.

When one studies this multiplicity of ideas and influences, it becomes apparent that the four models, which repeatedly emerge in this debate about the nature of archetypes, are as

- biological entities in the form of information which is hard-wired in the genes, providing a set of instructions to the mind as well as to the body
- organizing mental frameworks of an abstract nature, a set of rules or instructions but with no symbolic or representational content, so that they are never directly experienced
- core meanings which do contain representational content and which therefore provide a central symbolic significance to our experience
- metaphysical entities which are eternal and are therefore independent of the body.

In this book I hope to demonstrate that some of the confusion over the nature and meaning of the term 'archetype' arises when these concepts are not clearly distinguished from each other. Confusion arises, for example, when genetic instructions are also thought of as core symbolic meanings, when the two are actually quite different. On the one hand, genetic instructions contain no symbolic content and so cannot be the direct source of meaningful imagery. On the other hand, contemporary cognitive science is increasingly providing the empirical evidence to show that the human mind does contain core meanings which structure our perception of the world but these are built up from experience and are not innate or genetically specified, nor are they universal and eternal truths which exist independently of the human mind and brain (Schacter 1996; Dupré 2001).

If the term 'archetype' is used in so many different ways, which are mutually inconsistent, then it becomes too ambiguous a concept to have any value as a research tool for scientific investigation. The concept becomes no more than an interesting historical footnote in the empirical research literature and, until now, with few exceptions, this has been its fate in academic psychology. It has been seen as too vague, too varied in its definition and so too imprecise to be explored experimentally. This lack of precision has also produced widespread misconceptions among biologists and psychologists about Jung's ideas. Konrad Lorenz demonstrated such a misunderstanding when he described Jung's theory of the archetype as an inherited memory image, which he accordingly rejected – although he apparently later assured Marie-Louise von Franz that he did in fact accept Jung's theory of archetype in principle (von Franz 1975: 126–7). Contemporary biologists are often still under the impression that Jung was proposing the Lamarckian view that acquired characteristics could be inherited and that the collective unconscious is the repository of cumulative human experience.

As I have demonstrated, the ambiguity about archetypes can be traced directly back to Jung's own writing, in which he drew on philosophy, religion, mythology, physics, biology, psychology, psychiatry and psychoanalysis, and used these frames of reference to explore the concepts which might help him in his struggle to understand the nature and functioning of the human psyche. Each of these frameworks offered him one or other of the core themes which I have identified, and which provided him with a perspective through which to view the idea of archetype and define its essential features. Sometimes he wrote about archetypes as abstract organizing structures, sometimes as eternal realities, then again as core meanings; on other occasions, he adopted a very sophisticated ethological viewpoint, in which he identified archetypes as manifestations of instinct, a term which he used in a much more biologically accurate way than Freud. John Haule has highlighted these ambiguities and inconsistencies in Jung's use of the term archetypes and suggested that we can distinguish six meanings of the term (Haule 1999: 257). Some of his six categories are descriptive rather than conceptual (such as a description of the archetype as a numinous quality of experience) and my own view is that four categories are sufficient to differentiate the various core concepts of the archetype, concepts which were so frequently merged together in Jung's writings.

I can illustrate this merging of the four models, which I have identified with the following quotations, all taken from the same paragraph:

> Archetypes are by definition factors and motifs that arrange the psychic elements into certain images, characterized as archetypal, but in such a way that they can be recognized only by the effects they produce.

Here, Jung describes archetypes as organizing frameworks, which are not directly experienced, the second of the four models for the archetype which I have described. Jung then immediately continues:

> They exist pre-consciously, and presumably they form the structural dominants of the psyche in general.

In this phrase, Jung seems to suggest the third view of archetypes, that of core meanings, which provide a central symbolic significance to our experience. His next two sentences in this same paragraph add another perspective to the mixture:

> As *a priori* conditioning factors they represent a special psychological instance of the biological 'pattern of behaviour [which gives all things their specific qualities]. Just as the

manifestations of this biological ground plan may change in the course of development, so also can those of the archetype.

Jung's view here seems to merge the first model of archetypes as biological, genetic entities with the third model, that of predetermined meaning 'conditioning' our experience. Finally he says:

> Empirically considered, however, the archetype did not ever come into existence as a phenomenon of organic life, but entered into the picture with life itself.
>
> (Jung 1948[1942], note 2: para. 222)

This last sentence seems to suggest the fourth theme, in which archetypes are not biological entities but exist as a manifestation of eternal life; further evidence that this was sometimes Jung's view of archetypes can be found in another statement from a different paper:

> Whether this psychic structure and its elements, the archetypes ever 'originated' at all is a metaphysical question and therefore unanswerable.
>
> (Jung 1954[1938]: para. 187)

It does seem as though Jung did not differentiate clearly enough between these differing perspectives and probably did not see the need to do so. As he himself rather ruefully pointed out:

> I fancied I was working along the best scientific lines, establishing facts, observing, classifying, describing causal and functional relations, only to discover in the end that I had involved myself in a net of reflections which extend far beyond natural science and ramify into the fields of philosophy, theology, comparative religion and the humane sciences in general.
>
> (Jung 1954[1947]: para. 421)

It is probably futile to trawl painstakingly through Jung's *Collected Works*, finding evidence to suggest that one way of envisaging archetypes predominates over another in his writing. Neither Jung nor his early followers, such as Jolande Jacobi, saw the need to distinguish between these ways of conceptualizing archetypes.

Instead they seemed to feel that the fact that they found a variety of models for inherent or innate structures within the cultural, religious, philosophical, psychological and biological frameworks which they studied, provided cumulative evidence for the concept of the archetype. This kind of evidence suggests that one biographer of Jung, Frank McLynn, was fair to Jung in one respect, if not in others, in suggesting that Jung liked, as he put it, 'tacking between philosophy and biology', since this pre-empted the criticisms which would arise if he based the theory of archetypes too closely on models drawn from either discipline (McLynn 1996: 306). McLynn suggests that Jung feared being accused of Lamarckism if he concentrated too much on biological analogies; on the other hand, he may not have wished to be classified as a metaphysician, since this would undermine his claim that his theories had scientific status.

The state of knowledge of human information processing was not sufficiently developed for Jung and his supporters for them to recognize the significance of the crucial differences between the four themes which I have identified. They could not possibly have known, for example, that a contemporary cognitive science model of the human psyche would distinguish between two kinds of schema, one of which contains meaningful representational content, which is built up through learning and interaction with the external world, and is stored in the form of abstract and generalized patterns in implicit memory. The other kind of schema is a non-representational structure which contains no symbolic content, but which directs attention to crucial features in the environment.

Innate structures of the human mind cannot contain the symbolic and representational content which the idea of a core meaning requires, as Locke recognized, anticipating by over 300 years the work of contemporary philosophers and developmental psychologists (Locke 1689; Dupré 2001; Karmiloff-Smith 1992). In contrast, the kind of schema which is constructed in implicit memory contains core meanings which always result from a learning process. This will be discussed in more detail in Chapter 4. The evidence now available to us from contemporary cognitive science research would suggest that Jung was trying to reconcile models which are incompatible with each other in relation to the structures of the human psyche.

However, the failure to differentiate and choose between these conflicting models is not a position which contemporary analytical psychologists can continue to adopt. We do have access to the evidence provided by a modern, scientific conception of the functioning of the human mind, yet analytical psychologists often continue to fail to differentiate between one model of archetypes and another, apparently unaware of the theoretical inconsistencies which this approach creates. For example, we continue to fail to distinguish between implicit memory, which stores learnt information in an unconscious schematic format that provides us with core meanings, and innate inherited structures, which are hard-wired in the genes but which contain no symbolic content.

This distinction, which has emerged from scientific empirical research, between form, which can be inherited, and content, which cannot, had been anticipated many years ago in philosophy. In his discussion of the influence of Schopenhauer on Jung, Jarret (1999) writes:

> Interestingly, both authors specifically allow that Locke was right in his attack on innate ideas, since in his context 'ideas' are mental representations of material reality, and therefore can be learned only in experience. But they agree further that Locke overdogmatized in saying that nothing is innate. As Schopenhauer puts it, 'Locke goes too far in denying all innate truths inasmuch as he extends his denial even to our formal knowledge – a point in which he has been brilliantly rectified by Kant . . .' For Jung as for Schopenhauer the archetypes, the primordial images, the prototypical Ideas are the forms into which is poured the material content, with its individual and cultural qualities.
>
> (Jarrett 1999: 201)

Philosophical and scientific influences on the four themes which contribute to Jung's concept of the archetype

Before examining the new light which contemporary scientific research can shed on the nature of the archetype, I shall explore in this section the extent to which different frames of reference contributed to each of the four models interwoven in Jung's concept of the archetype. To recapitulate, these four models are:

- biological entities in the form of information which is hard-wired in the genes, providing a set of instructions to the mind as well as to the body
- organizing mental frameworks of an abstract nature, a set of rules or instructions but with no symbolic or representational content, so that they are never directly experienced
- core meanings which do contain representational content and which therefore provide a central symbolic significance to our experience
- metaphysical entities which are eternal and are therefore independent of the body.

Model 1: biological entities in the form of information which is hard-wired in the genes, providing a set of instructions to the mind as well as to the body

At first sight, this is the simplest approach to the concept of archetypes and it is the view which emerges in the research which examines the biological aspect of archetypal theory. Jung stated this view very clearly, writing that archetypes are 'inherited with the brain structure – indeed they are its psychic aspect' and

> The term archetype is not meant to denote an inherited idea, but rather an inherited mode of psychic functioning, corresponding to the inborn way in which the chick emerges from the egg, the bird builds its nest, a certain kind of wasp stings the motor ganglion of the caterpillar, and eels find their way to the Bermudas in other words it is a 'pattern of behaviour'.
>
> (Jung 1955: para. 1228)

However, problems soon begin to emerge, which Jung himself identified and which led to the distinction between the archetype-in-itself and the archetypal image. This distinction is clearly explained by Jacobi:

> The often cited comparison of the archetype with the Platonic eidos and the failure to distinguish between the non-perceptible 'archetype as such' and the perceptible, 'represented' archetype

have caused the archetypes to be regarded, in a manner of speaking, as inherited 'ready made images'. This has given rise to countless misunderstandings and unnecessary polemics.

(Jacobi 1959: 51)

The need for this distinction lies in the confusion over the characteristics of inherited psychic forms. When the model of the archetype as an inherited biological structure is linked with the model in which archetypes are seen to be organizing frameworks of an abstract nature, containing no representational content, then there is at first sight no incompatibility. Jacobi (1959: 52) points out: 'Jung's archetypes are a structural condition of the psyche, in which a certain constellation can bring forth certain "patterns" . . . this has nothing to do with the inheriting of definite images'. She is perfectly clear that archetypes are inherited possibilities of representation, hidden organizers of representations and that we can never be conscious of them as themselves, but only of the psychic material in which the archetypal pattern emerges and is expressed (Jacobi 1959: 52).

This link between the archetype as a biological inherited form and as an abstract organizing principle is strongly argued by Anthony Stevens (2002), when he describes archetypes as 'phylogenetically acquired, genome-bound units of information which programme the individual to behave in certain specific ways while permitting such behaviour to be adapted appropriately to environmental circumstances' (Stevens 2002: 60).

In spite of the apparent clarity offered by both Jacobi and Stevens, hints of ambiguity do emerge from time to time in their writings, which seem to suggest that they have slipped into linking archetypes as inherited entities with the third concept of archetypes as core meanings (which do have representational content). For example, Jacobi (1959) writes of archetypes as 'nuclei of meaning' and as typical motifs of the collective unconscious. She states that archetypes 'also embody ideations lying beyond the realm of the corporeal, metaphysical facts and factors, symbols etc, which are not included in the term "instinctive unconscious"' (Jacobi 1959: 61).

Although Stevens clearly differentiates between the archetype-as-such and the archetypal image, he then suggests that the former can be located in the limbic system of the brain and illustrates this with the mother–child archetypal system, a concept which suggest that the archetype-as-such contains specific representational content rather than being purely an 'innate neuropsychic potential' (Stevens 2002: 284–5). These issues will be investigated in more detail in Chapter 3.

For Jung, Jacobi and Stevens the archetype as an inherited entity is initially clearly linked to the concept of an abstract-organizing psychic structure; but then the distinction between the concept of an abstract, non-representational organizing structure and that of a core meaning is subtly lost, as the examples given previously show. This slippage is, in my view, the main cause of the suspicion or indifference which the academic world shows towards Jung's ideas of the collective unconscious and archetypes. As soon as there is a suggestion that core meanings can be inherited, then it begins to look as though information, which has been learnt through experience of the external world, can be passed on genetically because meaning implies a symbol and a symbol is a representation. Representations are formed only as a result of experience and it is therefore pure Lamarckism to suggest that representations can be inherited. This was clear even in Jung's day and he was at pains to refute this charge when he wrote 'It should on no account be imagined that there are such things as inherited ideas. Of that there can be no question' (Jung 1918: para. 14). However, the muddle remains in his writing as Hayman (1999: 228) demonstrates.

Some of the confusion over which aspects of the psyche are inherited can be traced back to the confusion between the two concepts which I shall examine next, first, that of abstract, non-representational organizing psychic structures, and second, of core representational, symbolic meanings. Other confusions arise furthermore even when model 1 of the archetype as a biological, inherited structure is linked to model 2 of the archetype as a content-less, organizing framework, an issue which I shall discuss in the next section.

Model 2: organizing mental frameworks of an abstract nature, a set of rules or instructions but with no symbolic or representational content, so that they are never directly experienced

This theme is identified clearly by Jacobi; she describes archetypes as hidden organizers of representations, a potential axial system, and uses a metaphor from chemistry to describe them as having the character of an invisible crystal lattice in solution (Jacobi 1959:

52). She goes on to link this idea of a content-less structure with the (then) newly emerging field of Gestalt theory; a Gestalt is a content-less form, a ground plan which retains its structure, regardless of the context in which it is expressed. The form itself is never directly experienced, but the underlying pattern organizes the material by which it becomes manifest. She gives the example of a simple melody which retains its fundamental pattern regardless of the key in which it is played, or the variations which are built on to it. At first sight this seems to be clear, but a pattern does imply a representational content, even if this is in the form of a purely mathematical description of its features. This begins to raise the question of whether an organizing structure can ever be entirely without representational content, whether model 2 can ever really be qualitatively distinguished from model 3, or only quantitatively. In the abstract, the idea of an irrepresentable organizing framework is attractive as a description of the archetype-as-such, but in practice, the examples which come to mind seem to contain elements, both of an organizing structure which cannot be directly experienced and of a core meaning which has representational content and hence, symbolic meaning.

A possible key to the source of this difficulty may lie in the influence on Jung of the philosophy of Immanuel Kant, who distinguished between noumena or 'concepts of pure reason', which cannot be experienced, and phenomena, which exist in the material world and so can be experienced. Hayman (1999) demonstrates that Jung blurred this distinction in a way that Kant would not have accepted, by regarding mental events, including fantasies, beliefs, dreams and hallucinations as empirically real and therefore classifying them as phenomena, even though they are not grounded in time or space. Brooke (1991: 75) concurs with this view, saying that Jung collapses Kant's distinction between noumena and phenomena, expanding the definition of the phenomenal world to include subjective psychological experience. De Voogd (1984) is even more succinct, saying that when Jung urges upon us the phenomenal reality of psychic manifestations, that in Kantian terms 'this amounts to nothing less than an invitation to regard the phenomenally unreal as the phenomenally real' (De Voogd 1984: 222). Bishop also takes Jung to task for an inadequate understanding of Kant's concept of the noumenon, criticizing him for the intellectual sleight of hand by which 'he pursued what we might call a strategy of "psychic relativism"' according to which he

redefined Kant's categories as a mere product of psychic functions'
(Bishop 2000: 182).

However, Jung did retain the view that the archetype-as-such
was content-less and the 'noumenon' is another concept from
which that of the archetype as a content-less organizing mental
structure is drawn. In the most thorough study to date of Jung's
Kantianism, De Voogd acknowledges this, saying 'something very
Kantian is going on when the irrepresentable archetype-as-such
is carefully distinguished from its visualizations in the form of
images and ideas or from instinctual self-perception' (De Voogd
1984: 226).

However, the temptation to combine model 1, of the archetype
as a biological predispostion, with model 2, in which it is thought
of as an abstract organizing structure, unknowable in itself, leads
us back into confusion. There is then an implied link between
Kant's philosophical distinction between noumenon and phenomenon and the biological distinction between genotype (inherited,
genetic instructions) and phenotype (the psychological and physical
features which express the genetic instructions). The genotype is
not the same thing as Kant's noumenon, nor is the phenotype
identical with his phenomenon. A thorough exploration of the
differences between these philosophical and the biological concepts
would take me away from my main task of identifying the various
frames of reference which contribute to the confusion over the
characteristics of archetypes; however, one point which illustrates
the difference is that a noumenon is immaterial, irrepresentable
and unknowable, while a genotype is a material structure, con-
sisting of particular sequences of DNA in our chromosomes.
The genotype cannot be experienced in itself, only in the
phenotype, but the genotype is a material reality, not a 'concept
of pure reason'.

The relationship between Plato's 'ideas' or 'pure forms' and
Jung's concept of the archetype is even more problematic than the
extent to which archetype-as-such and archetypal image can be
mapped onto Kant's concepts of noumenon and phenomenon.
Plato's 'pure form' provides one of the sources for the next concept
of the archetype, although it is significantly different from Kant's
noumenon. Bishop suggests that Jung failed to appreciate the
distinction between the Idea in the Platonic and the Kantian sense,
or chose to ignore the important differences between them (Bishop
2000: 160).

Model 3: core meanings which do contain representational content and which therefore provide a central symbolic significance to our experience

Jung acknowledged that he was influenced by Plato and at one point he said that the term archetype 'is an explanatory paraphrase of the Platonic eidos' (Jung 1954[1934]: para. 5). This word is literally translated as 'idea', but most Plato scholars consider that its meaning is more accurately represented by the word 'form'. However, Jung himself sticks to 'idea' and says that he uses the term to express: 'the formulated meaning of a primordial image by which it was represented symbolically'. He continues:

> the idea is a psychological determinant, having an *a priori* existence. In this sense, Plato sees the idea as a prototype of things, while Kant defines it as the 'archetype . . . of all practical employment of reason'.
>
> (Jung 1921: para. 732)

Jung does recognize here that Plato's 'ideas' (or forms) are not identical to Kant's noumena, which are irrepresentable and unknowable and so do not provide a core meaning. In contrast, Plato's forms are considered to be the real model of which all material reality is a derived copy and, as such, 'ideas' provide a core symbolic meaning to all experience. For example, Plato says that the 'form' of the good is 'the cause of all that is right and beautiful in all things' (Lindsay 1906: 210). Jung clearly considers archetypes to provide a core of symbolic meaning, saying:

> In Plato, however, an extraordinarily high value is set on the archetypes as metaphysical ideas, as 'paradigms' or models, while real things are held to be only copies of these model ideas.
>
> (Jung 1919: para. 275)

In his discussion of 'idea' in 'Definitions' (Jung 1921: paras 732–7) Jung explores Schopenhauer's development of Plato's 'idea'. Schopenhauer emphasized the visual aspect of the archetype, as Jung approvingly noted: 'For Schopenhauer the idea is a visual thing, for he conceives it entirely in the way that I conceive the primordial image'. It is therefore especially the philosophical concepts of Plato and Schopenhauer which most strongly contribute to this model of the archetype, in which it is seen to provide an *a priori* symbolic core of meaning to all experience. It is this model which seems to be uppermost when Jung writes about mandalas.

Model 4: metaphysical entities which are eternal and are therefore independent of the body

Another aspect of Plato's 'idea' or 'form' which seems to have been attractive to Jung is its eternal, transcendent quality: 'Take for instance the word "idea". It goes back to the eidos concept of Plato, and the eternal ideas are primordial images stored up . . . (in a supracelestial place) as eternal transcendent forms' (Jung 1954 [1934]: para. 68).

Jarrett explores the influence that Schopenhauer's thinking had on Jung, who was drawn to Schopenhauer's view that the mind can be extended beyond the world we perceive around us to the Platonic 'forms', and that the result is 'an enhancement of consciousness to the pure, will-less timeless subject of knowing' (Jarrett 1999: 197). Schopenhauer said that Plato's ideas 'always are, but never become nor pass away' (1958: para. 31).

In his preface to Jolande Jacobi's (1959) *Complex/Archetype/Symbol*, Jung makes it clear that he regards her as an authoritative exponent of his views on archetypes, and Jacobi also emphasizes their eternal quality. She investigates synchronicity in this light, linking this with archetypes which she regards as 'timeless, unlimited and the introspectively recognizable form of *a priori* psychic orderedness' (Jacobi 1959: 64). This transcendental aspect of the archetype is particularly emphasized by another of Jung's close circle, Liliane Frey-Rohn, who says that Jung conceived of the archetype as 'a primary model in the background of the psyche, which had its roots in the transcendental and non-psychic realm' (Frey-Rohn 1974: 96).

The new developments in physics which Jung discovered through his association with Wolfgang Pauli, the physicist and Nobel Prize winner, contributed to this model of the archetype as an acausal connecting principle. Jacobi says:

> For physics and psyche may be regarded as two aspects of the same thing, ordered according to a meaningful parallelism;

they are as it were, 'superimposed' the one on the other; they are 'synchronous' and, in their cooperation, not understandable on the basis of causality alone.

(Jacobi 1959: 64)

Jung used a series of coincidences to support his argument for synchronicity, as a principle operating outside space and time, and under Pauli's influence he began to use the language of quantum physics. Hayman says that 'Jung began to speak of the archetypes as having a "field of force" and to redefine them as transcendental arrangers of psychic forms inside and outside the psyche' (Hayman 1999: 407). Jung began to think of archetypes as manifestations of an absolute knowledge which is not accessible to consciousness, but probably is to the unconscious, under certain conditions.

It seems as though Jung was using quantum physics as supporting evidence for a model of archetypes as eternal and absolute realities, governed by different principles from those that operate in our world which is bounded by space and time. It may have appealed to him to bring together the latest scientific research in mathematics with the ancient concept of Platonic Forms – but attempting to bring these together in one framework with biology creates impossible theoretical conflicts.

Conclusions

The more we investigate the various strands which interweave in the concept of the archetype, the more evident it becomes that there are major tensions and contradictions between them, so much so that they can no longer all hold together as they could in Jung's day.

However, new insights on these models emerge from this study of the sources which have contributed to the various meanings of the term archetype. A biological model can be compatible with model 2, in relation to the archetype as a biologically emergent structure. Models 3 and 4 can never be innate because they are both concerned with the archetype as symbolically meaningful and representational, features which Darwinian theory defines as noninheritable because they are always formed from learnt or acquired experience. I am not claiming here that there is no such thing as transcendent reality, only that any sense we may have of it is never innate, and can be derived only from our experience of the real world around us, a position which echoes that of Jung in his dispute with Martin Buber when he wrote 'I make no transcendental statement. I am essentially empirical, as I have stated more than once. I am dealing with psychical phenomena and not with metaphysical assertions' (Jung 1963: 570; Stephens 2001). One problem for Jungian analysts is that the view of archetypes as transcendental and eternal realities which provide a core meaning has become the popular way in which they are understood. When non-analysts use the term 'archetypal' it usually seems to imply something akin to Plato's Pure Form and once a term has entered popular mythology in this way, it may be difficult for professionals to use it with a different, but more precise technical meaning.

A final issue of relevance is Jung's use of the concept of synchronicity to support his argument that archetypes are innate structures which allow us access to transcendental reality. His view was partly based on a misunderstanding of mathematical probabilities; he failed to appreciate that our sense that coincidences are meaningful is an illusion produced by the fact that non-conscious attention highlights certain chance occurrences precisely because they are meaningful to us. Statistically these coincidences have no significance, but humans do seem to have a poor intuitive sense of probabilities, with a marked tendency to underestimate the likelihood that two events will occur together by chance. Richard Dawkins (1998) gives a striking example from his own personal experience of the kind of coincidence which is often used as evidence of synchronicity. He chose a four digit combination for his bicycle lock one day and later received an authorization code for the academic office photocopier with exactly the same code. Dawkins points out that although the coincidence is impressive because the odds of matching all four digits of his bicycle combination are 1 in 10,000,

> There is no reason to suspect anything other than simple accident. The number of people in the world is so large compared with 10,000 that somebody, at this very moment, is bound to be experiencing a coincidence at least as startling as mine.
> (Dawkins 1998: 149)

Jung's concept of the archetypes as core meanings and as transcendental realities is based not only on a misunderstanding of mathematics but also on a distortion of biological principles. Symbols cannot be inherited, nor can genes be the vehicle for eternal truths. Genes are chemical structures, which interact with other chemical structures in the body and in that sense convey information which produces living organisms of incredible complexity. That is all they do. They cannot act as the carriers for any kind of complex symbolic information of the kind which is inherent in models 3 and 4. However, I do not agree with Carrette (1994) that the inconsistencies and ambiguities in the meaning of the word 'archetype' render it spurious and redundant. Instead I would suggest that it needs to be redefined, not as a cultural phenomenon as Pietikainen (1998) suggests, but as a psychological feature arising out of the development of the human brain. We do have to make a choice between a biological and a metaphysical view of archetypes and research developments in the biologically based fields of cognitive and developmental psychology also make it increasingly urgent for us to re-examine and update our biological concept of the archetype in the light of these discoveries. As Satinover (1985) wrote:

> We have learned from observation of infants that just as neither the mother nor the child is a *tabula rasa*, neither are they a predetermined lock and key. That is, the infant does not carry within an imago to project onto the adult, as we are accustomed to believe. Rather in the course of maturation, interactions between the mother and child alter them both. A fully developed pattern of behaviour is not inherited nor is it learned.
>
> (Satinover 1985: 82)

This developmental and interactive approach will underpin the exploration of the findings from research in other disciplines, which is the focus of Chapter 3.

Archetypes and image schemas

A developmental perspective

In Chapter 2, I showed how confusing the concept of the archetype becomes when we start to dissect the multiplicity of sources and meanings, which became woven together in Jung's own researches, and those of his close collaborators. I also showed that there are irreconcilable tensions between the various models of the archetype which Jung tried to bring together into a coherent whole, particularly in relation to the crucial question of whether any aspects of archetypes can be considered to be innate, genetically inherited structures.

In this chapter, I shall focus on contemporary developmental psychology research on the nature of innate structures in the human mind and take this aspect of the investigation of archetypes further. What does this research tell us about what is hard-wired into the human brain? How do the innate structures of the mind interact with the environment, and what psychic contents and processes emerge out of that interaction?

Innate processes in animals

The early ethological research of Nikolaas Tinbergen and Konrad Lorenz offered an instinct-based account of animal behaviour in which key environmental triggers would release specific innately determined responses in the animal under investigation. One of the most famous studies of these 'innate release mechanisms' was Lorenz's demonstration that greylag geese would imprint to any animal or human being that appeared in their field of vision immediately after hatching. Lorenz himself explained this behaviour as an expression of innate genetic instructions:

The gosling possesses innate information that, if translated into words, would read as follows: 'Whoever responds to your lost piping is your mother; take careful note of her appearance'. This first round of communication between mother and offspring constitutes the vital process of imprinting, which can never be repeated or reversed.

(Lorenz 1979: 146)

So how do ethologists understand the mechanisms behind these complex instinctual patterns of behaviour? What is the nature of the innate instructions which are activated by the 'right' environment? It is tempting to think that geese have some kind of innate template of the mother goose in their brains, which is triggered by the right match, but Lorenz's own research shows how mistaken this interpretation of the goose's behaviour would be. He found that 'when the dialogue takes place between a gosling and a human being, even if only a few times, it subsequently becomes apparent that the juvenile innate behaviour patterns of the freshly hatched gosling are permanently fixed on the human foster parent' (Lorenz 1979: 146). No one would possibly suggest that Konrad Lorenz's face would match some innate template of a mother goose.

Ethologists have also convincingly demonstrated that highly complex animal behaviour, which appears to show an intelligent mind at work is, in reality, the consequence of genetically programmed automatic responses to certain environmental triggers. It can easily be shown that the behaviour is mindless, in the sense that the animal does not have any long-term goal which is held in mind and which acts as a model, guiding the animal's behaviour. As Daniel Dennett has put it:

There are two profoundly different ways of building dams: the way beavers do and the way we do. The differences are not necessarily in the products but in the control structures within the brains that create them. A child might study a weaverbird building its nest and then replicate the nest herself . . . But it would be a big mistake to impute to the bird the sort of thought processes we know or imagine to be going on in the child. There could be very little in common between the processes going on in the child's brain and in the bird's brain. The bird is (apparently) endowed with a collection of interlocking special purpose minimalist subroutines, well designed

by evolution according to the notorious need-to-know principle of espionage: give each agent as little information as will
suffice for it to accomplish its share of the mission.

(Dennett 1995: 372)

However, as Dennett points out, this system works only when the
environment is regular and predictable enough for the automatic
sub-routines to produce the 'right' result. Natural selection makes
no allowance for the possibility that Konrad Lorenz may be the
first thing that a gosling sets eyes on after hatching. Very simple
experiments can demonstrate the inflexibility and automatic quality
of these innate behaviour routines and hence an animal's total
inability to modify them in response to a change in the environment. These kinds of experiments originated as a response to
George Romanes' suggestion that animals showed a capacity for
decision-making which showed an intelligent mind at work ([1882]
1904).

However, another early Darwinian, Conway Lloyd Morgan,
conducted much more rigorous experiments than Romanes did. He
observed a terrier learning to open a gate and showed that its
apparently intelligent actions did not arise from an understanding
of locks and levers, but originated in accidental movements as the
dog wildly pawed the gate in an attempt to get through. With
repetition the animal learnt which sequences of actions were effective and could open the gate, but without any understanding of the
principles underlying its learnt sequence of behaviour. Another
experiment looked at certain caterpillars which move from branch
to branch in search of foliage. The French naturalist Jean-Henri
Fabre placed a number of these caterpillars in a single file around
the neck of a vase one metre in circumference and observed them
for seven days as they followed each other round and round the
vase without stopping, behaviour which is clearly mindless in that
it would lead to certain death. Even simpler animals demonstrate
innate mechanisms which orientate them automatically towards
light; tube worms placed in a sea-water tank would build their
tubes at an angle directed towards the light, wherever the light was
placed. Experiments such as these clearly demonstrate the mindless
nature of the activity and how crucial it is that the characteristics
of the environment remain those in which the behaviour evolved
for that behaviour to provide an effective survival mechanism
(Sparks 1982: 12).

These simple automatic patterns of behaviour are algorithms, innate automatic sequences which have evolved by natural selection. As Dennett says:

> Here then is Darwin's dangerous idea: the algorithmic level *is* the level that best accounts for the speed of the antelope, the wing of the eagle, the shape of the orchid, the diversity of species, and all the other occasions for wonder in the world of nature. It is hard to believe that something as mindless and mechanical as an algorithm could produce such wonderful things. No matter how impressive the products of an algorithm, the underlying process always consists of nothing but a set of individually mindless steps succeeding each other without the help of any intelligent supervision; they are 'automatic' by definition; the workings of an automaton.
>
> (Dennett 1995: 56, original emphasis)

Innate structures of the human mind

The identification of what is innate is much simpler in relation to behavioural release mechanisms in animals than it is when we come to think about complex cognitive processes in humans.

Karl Marx, who knew Darwin's work and corresponded with him, had clearly grasped the key issue in relation to this distinction when he wrote:

> The spider carries out operations reminiscent of a weaver and the boxes which bees build could disgrace the work of many architects. But even the worst architect differs from the most able bee from the very outset in that before he builds a box out of boards he has already constructed it in his head. At the end of the work process he obtains a result which already existed in his mind before he began to build.
>
> (Marx 1995[1887]: 116)

The crucial distinction which Marx highlights in this remark is that humans have minds which are capable of creating and storing complex symbolic mental representations in a way which most animals are not. Animals may be capable of mental representation, but not the symbolic or propositional kind of representation that is demonstrated by human speech, writing and drawing. The distinction is probably best captured in Edelman's model of 'primary consciousness', which animals with certain brain structures possess, and higher order consciousness, probably unique to humans, which enables semantic and symbolic representation, an awareness of self and the ability to remember the past and imagine the future (Edelman and Tononi 2000: 202).

This brings us straight back to the problem: what is the precise nature of innate content as far as the human mind is concerned? Is the representational and symbolic functioning of the human brain another example of highly complex and apparently purposeful activity which can also be reduced to a series of mindless automatic algorithms? Do we deceive ourselves in thinking that our essential humanity lies in our consciousness, which overrides the automatic nature of animal behaviour and gives us a freedom of choice which other animals cannot exercise? The alternative view is that the human mind represents an evolutionary leap to a new level of biological organization, one that really does permit new, unpredictable outcomes to emerge from the interaction of genetic predisposition and environmental stimulus.

We have to turn to the research of developmental psychologists and cognitive scientists in order to begin to answer this question. To clarify the issues that their research investigates, I need to summarize two models which are at opposite ends of a theoretical spectrum and which offer fundamentally different accounts of the development of the range of cognitive capacities of the human mind.

Fodor's modularity or Piaget's tabula rasa

The infant mind as a tabula rasa

Piaget, who was analysed by Sabina Spielrein, was familiar with Jung's work on symbolism to which he referred (Vidal 2001). However, on the whole, Piaget rejected the idea that the infant mind contained any kind of innate knowledge. He viewed the brain as empty of any innate content and thought that knowledge could be acquired only by learning, through three processes, those of accommodation, assimilation and equilibration. As the infant's sensorimotor capacities develop and mature, knowledge of the world is organized by a general learning process. There are developmental stages which reflect milestones, or leaps forward, in an overall maturation process affecting all areas of psychological development including language, numeracy and spatial cognition.

Modularity

The alternative view of human cognitive development is that infants are pre-programmed to make sense of specific information sources. Each area of cognition, known as a domain, has its own developmental programme which is built on to innate specifications. The concept of modularity of mind was introduced by Fodor who argued that the mind is made up of 'genetically specified, independently functioning, special-purpose "modules" or input systems' (Karmiloff-Smith 1992: 2). Information from the environment is filtered through sensory transducers which transform the data into the right format for each special purpose module. These modules are encapsulated so that development and learning within one modular system does not influence the internal workings of another module (Fodor 1983).

An evolutionary perspective

The discipline of evolutionary psychology has emerged since the early 1990s as a development of the concept of modularity and as a reaction against Piaget's theory that the mind is a *tabula rasa* at birth. A succinct summary of the evolutionary basis of human activity as based on algorithms is the suggestion that

> various evolved social mentalities (e.g. information processing strategies and algorithms for care eliciting/seeking, caregiving/ providing, mate selection, alliance formation, and ranking behaviour) are the foundation stones for concept of self, systems of internal meanings (e.g. inner working models), role-taking behaviour, social signalling, self and other evaluation processes and a host of other crucial functions.
>
> (Bailey 2000: 54)

This approach is clear that mental functioning emerges from complex gene-environment interactions.

However, some key researchers in this field subscribe to a position in which a major part of human psychological functioning is considered to be innate and so by implication genetically determined and modular. Ranged on this side of the debate are cognitive scientists such as Steven Pinker (1997), Daniel Dennett (1995) and evolutionary psychologists such as Barkow, Cosmides and Tooby, whose book *The Adapted Mind* (1992) has greatly influenced an evolutionary perspective on human psychological functioning.

For example, Steven Pinker (1994) has concluded that language is a form of innate instinctual knowledge which is hard-wired into the human brain and draws on this to suggest that:

> If language, the quintessential higher cognitive process, is an instinct, maybe the rest of cognition is a bunch of instincts too – complex circuits designed by natural selection, each dedicated to solving a particular family of computational problems posed by the ways of life we adopted millions of years ago.
>
> (Pinker 1994b: 97)

Pinker suggests that the key characteristic of these inbuilt instincts is that they are a genetic store of the kind of information which our ancestors needed to have to survive. He suggests that they include, for example, an intuitive knowledge of mechanics, giving us an innate understanding of the forces that move objects and a capacity to identify danger, such as might be posed by heights or predatory animals. However, Pinker (1997) also suggests that more abstract patterns may be stored as innate algorithms, such as concepts of justice, a sense of self and patterns of kinship within a family.

Unfortunately, these views held by some cognitive scientists about the innate aspects of the human psyche demonstrate a surprisingly similar confusion to that which we find among analytical psychologists in relation to the degree to which archetypes can both be inherited and contain symbolic representational content. The algorithms which Pinker proposes seem to contain core meanings and the question remains unanswered as to how these can be reconciled with the characteristics of inherited genetic instructions, since symbolic meaning cannot be passed on through the genes. The genetic infrastructure (30,000 genes) is too small by far to encode the infinite range of symbols that the human mind can produce in the course of one day, let alone in a lifetime.

The crucial question which is raised by the model offered by these authors concerns the nature of the information contained in these postulated genetic programmes. Are they, like behavioural algorithms in animals, programmed sequences of automatic behaviour or attention which are triggered by a particular environmental stimulus? If so, what is the relationship between these automatic genetically programmed patterns of behaviour and the conceptual and symbolic aspects of the situation they relate to? If an algorithm for caregiving is triggered by the sight of one's own infant, does this algorithm include information about concepts such as helplessness, dependence, attachment? If so, how have symbolic semantic concepts become stored in a package of genetic instructions? Symbolic meaning cannot be inherited because it consists of representations which are the result of learning about the world and the product of cortical rather than sub-cortical activity; it is pure Lamarckism to suggest that these symbolic meanings can then be inherited. This kind of inherent contradiction in the algorithmic model which Pinker, Dennett and others offer as an explanation for human psychological functioning is not explored in their respective publications and one wonders if they have even recognized that the problem exists.

New developmental models

There is another theoretical framework for understanding human cognitive development, one which has emerged out of the debate between modularity and constructivism and which has succeeded in combining features of both these opposing viewpoints into a rich dialectical synthesis. One of the foremost centres for investigating this 'third way' was the Medical Research Council's Cognitive Development Unit at University College London, out of which emerged much of the research that I discuss. John Morton, Mark H. Johnson, Annette Karmiloff-Smith and others propose a developmental model in which the innate content of the infant mind consists mainly of initial predispositions and attention biases which activate learning.

This model thoroughly investigates the crucial question of the mode of functioning of our genes and challenges the assumption that a genetic code contains complex psychological information which is activated by an environmental stimulus. Karmiloff-Smith makes this point quite explicit:

> The brain is not prestructured with ready-made representations; it is channelled to progressively *develop* representations

via interaction with both the external environment and its own internal environment. And as I stressed above, it is important not to equate innateness with presence at birth or with the notion of a static genetic blueprint for maturation. Whatever innate component we invoke, it becomes part of our biological potential only through interaction with the environment; it is latent until it receives input.

(Karmiloff-Smith 1992: 10, original emphasis)

The interactionist model for biological development proposed by these developmental psychologists requires a fundamental and vital shift in our view of innate mental content. It is easy to assume that the term 'innate' means that there is information stored in a genetic code waiting, like a biological Sleeping Beauty, to be awakened by the kiss of an environmental Prince. This apparently common-sense view of innateness is frequently implicit in discussion about archetypes, in Jung's own writing and in that of many former and contemporary analytical psychologists. The concept that genetic codes contain a blueprint of complex information has a great deal in common with the view that archetypes are biological entities that also contain a core meaning.

It is a model which is hard for non-scientists to abandon because it seems to offer a simple and clear explanation of the role of innate structures in the human psyche. Furthermore, many evolutionary psychologists seem to have fallen into the same trap; although they have shown no interest at all in examining the parallels between their own concepts of innate, modular, algorithms and Jung's model of archetypes, there are many similarities between them. One such similarity is the mistaken assumption that information is contained in some form, however abstract and schematized, in the genes and that the environment activates and gives detailed embodied expression to that stored abstract potential. However, a developmental perspective reveals the flaws in this logic. As Elman et al. (1999) write:

The blueprint view of the genome, in which the genetic material somehow contains a literal image of the target animal is easy to reject. Nothing remotely resembling such a blueprint has ever been discovered. Nor is such a blueprint even logically possible, since there is simply not enough space in the genome to contain a full and complete description of the adult. Those animals in which there is, if not a blueprint, a straightforward and relatively direct relationship between genome and phenotype (as in mosaic species such as the nematode C. Elegans) arguably represent the upper bound of complexity which is possible given this sort of a tight genetic control on development.

(Elman *et al.* 1999: 350)

The recently completed map of the human genome offers conclusive evidence for the accuracy of these comments. Instead of the 100,000 or more genes which scientists expected to find, there are no more than about 30,000 in the human genetic code. It would be impossible for the complexity of a human being, both body and mind, to be stored as a blueprint of information in such a small number of genes.

The role of genetic instructions: the gene as catalyst

The view of genes which emerges from this developmental perspective is that of the gene as a catalyst. The key distinction from the model of the gene as blueprint is that the gene as a catalyst contains no information in isolation (Elman *et al.* 1999: 351–61).

However, the gene as a catalyst is highly interactive with the environment – how does this come about, if the gene does not have informational content? Developmental psychologists suggest that the answer probably lies in the distinction between process and content; there needs to be an innately specified mechanism of analysis, not necessarily innately specified content (Karmiloff-Smith 1992: 42).

The innate component could be as simple as a mechanism for focusing attention on to specific perceptual patterns, just as it seems to be in many animals. These patterns can then be stored in a simple schematized form, which then allows all similar patterns to be recognized. It is important to point out that it is not the case that the schematized pattern itself is stored as information in the genes, but rather, that the algorithm for focusing attention on to a particular pattern of information is activated by certain highly specific stimuli. In gulls, it is the red spot beneath the mother's beak which arouses this interest (Sparks 1982: 212). The obvious example of a similar process in humans is the infant's attention to and recognition of the basic pattern of the human face from the earliest weeks of life. Human infants do not have a model of the human face stored in their genes, but they do have genetic instructions (algorithms) to pay particular attention to any face-like pattern which appears in their visual field, and this is the only innate information that is required.

This leads us onto the experiments that have conclusively demonstrated the existence of specific attentional mechanisms in infants of a few weeks. One of the most thoroughly investigated of these is that of attention to the human face. Johnson and Morton (1991) conducted a range of experiments on newborn human infants to evaluate whether face recognition is innately specified. They showed these infants head-shaped boards with black features, some of which had the arrangement of the human face and others with alternative patterns. A crucial part of this research demonstrated that newborn infants were far more interested in watching a face-like image than any of the other options.

Their conclusion is that 'infants are born with some knowledge concerning the visual structure of the human face' (Johnson and Morton 1991: 103). They have called this mechanism 'Conspec' because it is the means whereby newborn infants recognize the conspecifics of their own species, the pattern of the human face. It does not allow differentiation between individual faces, such as the mother's or father's. The latter is a learning process, based on other mechanisms, that emerges some weeks later and depends on Conspec only to the extent that Conspec ensures that the baby will pay sufficient attention to human faces.

It would be easy to fall, once again, into the trap of concluding that the basis for Conspec must be an explicit representational image of the human face that somehow innately pre-exists in the human mind, enabling the meaning of human faces to be recognized. However, 'knowledge' does not have to mean this; innate knowledge can include the body's predetermined reactions to certain stimuli, and the key feature of Conspec is that it causes the infant to turn its gaze and attention towards the specific stimulus of the human face. Johnson and Morton suggest that this may be its only function and state that:

> It should be clear that we believe that young infants orient to faces under the guidance of a sensory motor reflex; the newborn does not require to understand the 'meaning' of a face.

That is to say, there is nothing social or intentional in the newborn's preferential orienting toward faces.

(Johnson and Morton 1991: 141)

Johnson and Morton suggest that all that may be required is a
subcortical mechanism which orientates the infant's attention
towards any face-like object in the periphery of its visual field.
Since the object which most commonly appears in this place is the
mother's face, Conspec could ensure that the infant is given plenty
of opportunity to learn the characteristics of the mother's face,
without the need to postulate innate representations of faces.

These sophisticated experiments provide crucial support for the
view that innate structures do not contain symbolic propositional
content but are simple stimulus response sequences, processed at a
sub-cortical level, which ensure that the infant's attention turns to
the key features in its environment that are essential for its
psychological as well as physical development.

This model is also strongly supported by the international collaborative research group I have already extensively quoted, which
state that:

> some innate predispositions – architectural, chronotopic and,
> rarely, representational – channel the infant's attention to
> certain aspects of the environment over others. Our view is
> that these predispositions play different roles at different levels,
> and that as far as representation-specific predispositions are
> concerned, they may only be specified at the subcortical level
> as little more than attention grabbers so that the organism
> ensures itself of a massive experience of certain inputs prior to
> subsequent learning. As we will argue throughout the book, at
> the cortical level, representations are not pre-specified: at the
> psychological level representations *emerge* from the complex
> interactions of brain and environment and brain systems
> among themselves.

(Elman *et al.* 1999: 108, original emphasis)

The profound implications of their work for Jungian theory have
been recognized by several analytical psychologists (Hogenson
2001; McDowell 2001). In particular this model refutes any possibility of innate (genetically specified) archetypal imagery, as I will

explore later. First, however, I will describe the current state of knowledge about the developmental processes which build upon these genetically specified orientating mechanisms and which then begin to organize the mass of information which bombards the senses of the newborn infant.

The brain as a self-organizing structure: an interactionist model for human psychological development

If core meanings can never be innate, if complex symbolic information cannot be contained in the genes which are passed on from parent to child, a new framework is needed for understanding the psychological development of the human infant. We need to explain the fact that we almost all develop the crucial skills of language, numeracy, reasoning, a sense of identity, a capacity for empathic relationship with others and, central to all these, the capacity to symbolize, so that we acquire a sense that experience is meaningful.

The principle of self-organizing emergent properties of the human mind is rapidly gaining ground over a more genetically deterministic model (Dupré 2001; Elman *et al.* 1999; Jaffe *et al.* 2001; Sander 2002; Schore 1994; Stern 1985; Tronick 2002). Developmental research supports the view that new meaning is constantly being created as a central part of the process of psychological development.

A crucial feature of this process is that it is highly sensitive to and dependent on the interpersonal environment; the infant's caregivers play a vital role in adapting their responses to the infant's constantly changing developmental needs. Pioneering empirical research confirms this view. For example, Sander (2002) suggests that development depends on the

> negotiation of a sequence of increasingly complex tasks of adaptation or 'fitting together', between the infant and its caregiving environment over the first years of life. This is a sequence of negotiations of connectedness in the interactions between infant and mother that constructs the bridge to organization at the psychological level.
>
> (Sander 2002: 13)

Sander argues that each living system – each organism – thus is seen as self-organizing, self-regulating and self-correcting within its surround, its environment. Furthermore, he suggests that we can identify principles in the process of exchange between organism and its context of life support that are present at all levels of complexity in living systems, from the cellular to the organization of consciousness. The principles that he highlights are those of specificity, rhythmicity, recurrence and pattern to coherence, wholeness and unity in the organization of component parts. Sander (2002) provides powerful support for this view with a remarkable experiment in which one group of neonates was fed on demand compared with another group who were fed every four hours regardless of their state. The results were remarkable. Within a few days, the demand-fed sample began to show the emergence of one or two longer sleep periods in each 24 hours and, after a few more days, these longer sleep periods began to occur more frequently at night, in contrast to the neonates fed every four hours who showed no such change. In other words, the sleep rhythms of the demand-fed infants began to synchronize with the diurnal 24-hour day of the caregiver. Sander concludes:

> The appearance of a new and continuing 24-hour circadian rhythmicity in the demand-fed infant–caregiver system can be seen as an emergent property of a system in a state of stable regulation. The infant becomes a system within a larger system, held together by the capability of biorhythms to phase-shift, increase or decrease period length, moving in or out of synchrony with other rhythms.
>
> (Sander 2002: 24)

Jaffe *et al.* (2001) also offer evidence of vocal rhythm coordination between infant and adults in support of the crucial role that rhythm plays in the moment-by-moment adaptations between infant and caregiver. They showed that the coordination of inter-personal timing involves the prediction of each partner's timing pattern from that of the other and that vocal rhythm coordination at age 4 months predicts attachment and cognition at 12 months. This capacity for rhythmic coordination is thus seen as essential to cognition and bonding.

This developmental process also underpins the emergence of complex symbolic representations out of the self-organization of the human brain, in the context of relationships. It is the model which clearly emerges in attachment theory, another field of study that is revolutionizing the theory and practice of all modalities of psychotherapy. The central research tools of attachment theory, the Strange Situation and the Adult Attachment Interview, show how internal working models store accumulated experience of early relationships into patterns of meaning which determine a person's attitudes and behaviour to their subsequent relationships. Allan Schore (1994) has investigated, in extraordinary detail, the research evidence that underpins an interactionist framework within which the intense relationships of early life directly influence the development of key parts of the brain. He writes:

> The mechanism of imprinting, a very rapid form of learning which underlies attachment bond formation, has been understood to involve an irreversible stamping of early experience upon the developing nervous system.
>
> (Schore 1994: 116)

For example, he offers evidence that the mother's face is an arousal generating cue for attachment behaviour and that this effect is produced by direct stimulation of the dopaminergic pathways of the orbito-frontal cortex (Schore 1994: 117). Schore offers further evidence that leads him to conclude that the right hemisphere is the repository of Bowlby's unconscious internal working models of the attachment relationship (Schore 2000b).

However, this account of the neurological mechanisms that underpin self-organization in the human brain needs to be complemented by an analysis of the information processing and the mental models to which those neurological processes give rise. The key processes and stages involved in the developmental aspects of human information-processing are gradually being identified by cognitive scientists. Jean Mandler (1992), for example, has described the earliest, primitive cognitive structures, image schemas, that are formed in the early days and weeks of a baby's life. An international collaboration between cognitive scientists and developmentalists in San Diego, Pittsburgh, London, Oxford and Rome has identified the characteristics of the self-organizing processes that build upon the basis of these image schemas, stimulating the development of ever more complex representations and forms of knowledge (Elman et al. 1999). Some cognitive scientists are finding evidence that information is repeatedly reanalysed and re-encoded into ever more complex forms of representation, in pace with the increasing cognitive capacities of the human brain during the course of development. One such mechanism has been identified by Karmiloff-Smith as 'representational redescription', a process of repeated recoding of stored information into new formats which eventually results in representations that can become conscious and expressed in language.

These two features, image schemas and representational redescription, will now be described in more detail.

Image schemas

Mandler drew a crucial distinction between perceptual recognition and perceptual analysis. Perceptual recognition is a sensorimotor activity which takes place automatically and does not require any conceptual framework. Mandler writes:

> We should not be misled by the complexity of these perceptual processing mechanisms. They are sophisticated, of course, but then so are the perceptual processing mechanisms of most organisms, or, for that matter, the industrial vision machines that neatly discriminate nuts from bolts. To categorize incoming stimuli into different types is a basic component of a perceptual recognition device; by itself, this ability tells us nothing about the formation of accessible concepts that may be used for the purposes of thought and reflection. The industrial machine may throw nuts into one bin and bolts into another (making its choices by, for example, computing the ration of the diameter of each object to its perimeter), but we would not want to say that it has a concept of nuts and bolts.
>
> (Mandler 1988: 117)

These procedural skills are just as much in evidence in other animals as in humans and are the automatic outcome of the genetically determined 'algorithms' described by Dennett and others.

However, Jean Mandler has convincingly argued that there is another process in operation in the earliest stages of infant life, that of perceptual analysis. She suggests that this is an active process of comparison between stimuli, which is the earliest evidence of a contemplative attitude and that this constitutes the basis of concept formation. She proposed that the first step on the conceptual organizational ladder is the formation of 'image schemas'. These are the earliest and most primitive form of representation in that they are conceptual structures mapped from spatial structures. Primitive conceptual knowledge takes a very different form from the complex symbolic knowledge of later life. It can be shown experimentally that very small babies demonstrate some kind of grasp of basic physical laws; at 3 months they show surprise if two solid objects seem to occupy the same space and at 4 months, if a solid object appears to have passed through a solid surface. However, this does not necessarily mean that babies have an innate complex conceptual knowledge of the laws of physics. One of the foundations of the conceptualizing capacity is the image schema in which spatial structure is mapped into conceptual structure.

Image schemas are notions such as PATH, UP-DOWN, CONTAINMENT, FORCE, PART-WHOLE, and LINK notions that are thought to be derived from perceptual structure. For example, the image schema PATH is the simplest conceptualization of any object following any trajectory through space, without regard to the characteristics of the object or the details of the trajectory itself. According to Lakoff and to Johnson, image schemas lie at the core of people's understanding, even as adults, of a wide variety of objects and events and of the metaphorical extensions of these concepts to more abstract realms. They form, in effect, a set of primitive meanings.

(Mandler 1992: 591)

Mandler gives an example of the concept of animacy and of the part image schemas might play in its formation. She suggests that the image schemas of PATH and LINK constitute the core meanings, so that 'a first concept of animals might be that they are objects that follow certain kinds of paths, that begin motion in a particular way, and whose movement is often coupled in a specific fashion to the movement of other objects' (Mandler 1992: 591). There is evidence to show that from an early age, infants can recognize self-motion, which characterizes animal movement (Leslie 1988).

Image schemas would therefore seem to have certain key features that are similar to some of the ways in which Jung conceptualized archetypes and this will be discussed in more detail below. First, I will explain the process of representational redescription.

Representational redescription

Image schemas are the first stage of a process whereby the brain constantly sorts and classifies sensory information into meaningful conceptual categories. The process itself has been called 'representational redescription' and it offers a precise account of the self-organizing processes out of which new cognitive structures and functions emerge, building on the foundation of image schemas.

In this model, information is constantly recoded into a different format, initially in each domain and then into representations that can be used across domains; in other words, knowledge acquired in one area of learning becomes available for use in other areas only when a certain level of representation of information has been achieved. This developmental process may proceed at different rates in different domains, so that a child who has reached a certain level of representation in the domain of language may be functioning at a different level of representation in the domain of numeracy.

At the first level, representations are in the form of procedures for analysing and responding to stimuli in the external world. These are implicit representations and they cannot be used across domains but are only available for processing within each domain of knowledge. These level-1 representations are procedures that remain in a child's mind and may be drawn on at any time for rapid automatic processing.

The next stage involves the formation of conceptual (not procedural like level-1) representations that encode the generalized themes available in information from the external world. They map the similarities between different types of information; for example, the concept of a zebra as a striped animal, a process that then allows the analogy to be made between the animal and a zebra crossing. These level E-1 (E for explicit) representations can be related to other representations and so allow learning in one domain to be drawn on in another. This is also the case for the next two levels of representation.

However, E-1 representations are not available to conscious access and verbal report. In contrast, at the next level, E-2 representations are available to consciousness but not yet in verbal form. They remain in the form of spatial, kinaesthetic representations, allowing us to draw diagrams of the information they contain even though we may not be able to express the concepts in language. Finally at level E-3, knowledge can be expressed in language. Verbal accounts can be given of the knowledge contained in these representations.

As Karmiloff-Smith says: 'This pervasive process of representational redescription gives rise to the manipulability and flexibility of the human representational system' (Karmiloff-Smith 1992: 186). It is a process that allows knowledge to become increasingly accessible to different parts of the cognitive system, so that consciousness itself can be seen to be an emergent property of the constantly reiterated process of representational redescription.

Representational redescription and Fordham's model of deintegration and reintegration

Karmiloff-Smith's developmental model has some similarities with the deintegration reintegration process that Michael Fordham proposed to account for the psychological development of the human infant. He wrote:

> In essence, deintegration and reintegration describe a fluctuating state of learning in which the infant opens itself to new experience and then withdraws in order to reintegrate and consolidate those experiences.
>
> (Fordham 1988: 64)

This sounds very similar to phases of representational redescription, where an initial phase, in which the infant's attention is focused on external stimuli, is followed by a second phase in which attention becomes focused on the changes in the newly formed representations in the infant's mind, so that they can eventually become conscious and expressible in imagery and language. Fordham's model also has some similarities with Piaget's concept of assimilation

However, there would seem to be some fundamental differences in that Fordham's model describes emotional as well as cognitive development and, at first sight, the representational redescription model seems to be a solely cognitive model. This argument can be countered to some extent by the evidence that shows that representational redescription is also the process that underpins the child's development of a theory of mind, the capacity to experience oneself and others as emotional beings with beliefs, desires and intentions (Karmiloff-Smith 1992: 134). The cognitive processing of emotion is as vital a part of an emotional experience as physiological arousal and an account of the mechanisms that allow that capacity to develop adds to our understanding of the formation of a sense of identity. Representational redescription would seem to be a vital part of the gradual formation of a sense of self and of a capacity to relate emotionally to other people. This is entirely compatible with Fordham's view that, for the human infant, 'individuation becomes the realization of his condition through the development of self-representations' (Fordham 1985: 54).

The concept of the self

Another feature of Fordham's model which is not found in the account of representational redescription described by Karmiloff-Smith (1992) is that of the original or primary self. Fordham suggested that the primary self was 'integrated, a psychosomatic potential waiting to unfold in interaction with the environment' (Astor 1995: 53). At first sight, this contrasts with the view of the self offered by developmental psychologists such as Daniel Stern (1985), who suggested that the self is an emergent product of development, not an a priori structure. However, once again we can reconcile these positions by considering the self to be an abstract concept, a way of conceptualizing all the possible emergent features of the human mind, both those that are realized in development and those that are not; this would be the logical conclusion of Fordham's statement that the self is a psychosomatic potential.

Archetypes re-examined in the light of developmental research

This explosion of developmental research on the brain offers analytical psychologists exciting new frameworks within which we can investigate the nature of archetypes. If we fail to examine the concept of archetypes in the light of this research, we run the risk that it will become an outdated irrelevance which no one takes seriously but ourselves. However, this research also presents us with difficult choices in identifying which of these perspectives most accurately captures the essential features and flavour of the concept of archetypes, as Jung originally described them and as analytical psychologists use the concept today. The task is rendered even more complicated by the conceptual over-determination that permeated Jung's writing about archetypes, which I have explored in Chapter 2.

If we now return to the four models of archetypes that I identified in Chapter 1 we can re-evaluate them in the light of the developmental research I have been exploring in this chapter, and examine the extent to which they are compatible with the evidence that emerges from such research, thus clarifying their accuracy or otherwise in biological, and developmental terms.

The four models that are implicit (and sometimes explicit) in Jung's concept of archetypes are:

- biological entities in the form of information which is hard-wired in the genes, providing a set of instructions to the mind as well as to the body
- organizing mental frameworks of an abstract nature, a set of rules or instructions but with no symbolic or representational content, so that they are never directly experienced
- core meanings which do contain representational content and which therefore provide a central symbolic significance to our experience
- metaphysical entities which are eternal and are therefore independent of the body.

Model 1: biological entities in the form of information which is hard-wired in the genes, providing a set of instructions to the mind as well as to the body

The developmental view of genes that I have outlined considers them to be catalysts rather than blueprints. Genes can contain sets of instructions, but they are very simple subcortical routines that are sufficient to kick-start a developmental process. Genes do not and cannot contain detailed information about the mental products that might emerge out of that developmental process because they contain no symbolic representational information at all.

This model of the role of genes in psychological development has considerable implications for analytical psychology in relation to the concept of archetypes. If the only role of genes in psychological development is the minimalist function of acting as a catalyst, it eliminates any possibility of viewing archetypes as hard-wired structures containing genetic knowledge that guides development. There can be no such innate 'knowledge' of universal themes because this kind of knowledge is the product of cortical functioning, which is never genetically predetermined. Analytical psychologists who adhere to this model of archetypes do so against an increasing tide of evidence about the developmental processes that guide the emergence of the sense of psychological meaning. It is time to abandon the concept of archetype as a form of innate, genetically transmitted knowledge.

Model 2: organizing mental frameworks of an abstract nature, a set of rules or instructions but with no symbolic representational content, so that they are never directly experienced

A developmental analysis demonstrates that this model of archetypes is compatible with the earliest forms of implicit representations – the image schemas which form the first stage in the representational redescription process by which the mind creates conscious thoughts, words and images.

These earliest representations can never become explicit because they exist in a schematic and procedural format. Cause and effect may be connected in these very early representations, enabling an infant, for example, to recognize the difference between the self-propelled movement shown by living creatures and movement of an inanimate object. However, these early implicit representations do not contain the complex symbolic concepts that develop through the process of representational redescription and that form the basis of the older child's capacity to recognize and describe an animal in words or pictures. These primitive representations are non-propositional and cannot contain explicit symbolic content.

This model of the archetype is therefore compatible in some respects with developmental research on the nature of early non-propositional representations. However, it is crucial to recognize that, even at this very early stage, these image schemas, the earliest representational models of the world that begin to be constructed in the infant's mind, are not innate, but already reflect a considerable degree of learning. The pattern of learning is nearly identical for all children because certain key features of the environment that the child's attention is focused on remain constant across all cultures. The laws of motion that determine the movement of physical objects remain the same in China and the USA. The same is true of infants' experience of their mouth sucking on their mother's nipple.

If we adopt this model for archetypes, we have to discard the view that they are genetically inherited and consider them to be reliably repeated early developmental achievements. However, this view of archetypes initially appears to restrict their content largely to primitive representations of the physical properties of the environment, which form a crucial foundation for our understanding of the world but can never become conscious. The concept of archetypal imagery would then become meaningless in this context and archetypes would cease to have any real value as vehicles for conveying symbolic meaning or as analytic tools. Indeed McDowell has specifically criticized the image schema model for archetypes on the grounds that it restricts archetypes to a few limited abstract concepts (McDowell, *Journal of Analytical Psychology* Internet discussion 2002).

However, the concept of image schemas is much richer than this. It was adopted by developmentalists, such as Jean Mandler, from its original use by the cognitive linguists, Lakoff and Johnson, who suggest that 'image schemas lie at the core of people's understanding, even as adults, of a wide variety of objects and events and *of the metaphorical extensions of these concepts to more abstract realms*' (quoted in Mandler 1992: 591, my emphasis). Image schemas form the basis of polysemy, which is 'the extension of a central sense of a word to other senses by devices of the human imagination, such as metaphor and metonymy' (Johnson 1987: xii).

The image schema would therefore seem to be a model that, for the first time, offers a developmentally sound description of the archetype-as-such and of the archetypal image. The abstract pattern itself, the image schema, is never experienced directly, but acts as a foundation or ground plan that can be likened to the concept of the archetype-as-such. This provides the invisible scaffolding for a whole range of metaphorical extensions that can be expressed in conscious imagery and language and that would therefore seem to correspond to the archetypal image. These metaphorical elaborations are always based on the Gestalt of the image schema from which they are derived.

In *The Body in the Mind* Johnson (1987) investigates systematically this process whereby image schemas are metaphorically extended from the physical to the non-physical realm. He suggests that 'it is a central claim of "cognitive grammar" that metaphorical projections of this sort are one of the chief means for connecting up different senses of a term'. For example, he says:

> [T]he OUT schema which applies to spatial orientation is metaphorically projected onto the cognitive domain where there are processes of choosing, rejecting, separating, differentiating abstract objects, and so forth. Numerous cases, such as *leave out, pick out, take out,* etc. can be either physical bodily actions that involve orientational schemata, or else they can be metaphorically orientated mental actions. What you *pick out* physically are spatially extended objects; what you *pick out* metaphorically are abstract mental or logical entities. But the relevant preconception schema is generally the same for both senses of *picking out*.

(Johnson 1987: 34, original emphases)

I am indebted to David Rosen for drawing my attention to a cognitive science article which examines Haiku poetry. Blasko and Merski (1998) suggest that the combination of simplicity of form and profoundness of meaning emerges out of the bodily basis of metaphor. They argue that if image schematic perceptual experiences play a role in cognitive organization, then conventional metaphorical mappings should be reflected in our language and in our poetry.

The image schema is a mental Gestalt, developing out of bodily experience and forming the basis for abstract meanings. Image schemas are the mental structures which underpin our experience of discernible order, both in the physical and in the world of imagination and metaphor.

My own view, explored in a previous article, is that the image schema meets many of the requirements for a contemporary developmental model of the archetype (Knox 1997). Kotsch (2000) has also adopted this approach to the concept of the archetype. While image schemas are without content in themselves, they provide a reliable scaffolding on which meaningful content is organized and constructed, thus meeting the need for a model that provides for the archetype-as-such and the archetypal image. In Chapter 1, I questioned Stevens' suggestion that there might be discrete archetypes, such as the mother archetype, on the grounds that this model requires too much representational content. 'Mother' is a concept but the image schema of 'containment' the bodily experience of being held and the accompanying physiological sensations of warmth, comfort and security, are not initially symbolic although they become so with the metaphorical elaboration of the image schema.

Model 3: core meanings which do contain representational content and which therefore provide a central symbolic significance to our experience

In a detailed study of the evolutionary concepts that informed Jung's psychological models, Hogenson (2001) has highlighted the rapid shift that is taking place, away from the 'Chomskian' paradigm that presupposes genetic encoding of knowledge (such as the syntactical rules governing language), towards a model in which it is the learning processes by which the brain categorizes information that can be considered to be innate. Hogenson (2001: 607) concurs with Saunders and Skar (2001), suggesting that 'archetypes are the emergent properties of the dynamic developmental system of brain, environment and narrative'. As core meanings they cannot be considered innate in the sense of 'hardwired' but could be considered to be a form of self-organizing emergent structure.

The difficulty that arises with this approach is the suggestion that Saunders and Skar (2001) make that archetypes cease to be differentiated from complexes, indeed they become a special category of complex. The real problem is that complexes contain unconscious symbolic information, thoughts, emotions, beliefs which share a central emotional theme. Complexes would therefore seem to contain considerable information in the form of symbolic representations; and the problem with viewing archetypes in this way is that they lose a key distinguishing characteristic, that of the archetype-as-such as a primitive sketch or Gestalt without information or representational content.

Model 4: metaphysical entities which are eternal and are therefore independent of the body

At first sight, a developmental approach cannot be integrated with this model of archetypes, which derives largely from Plato's 'ideas' or true forms. Whether there are eternal, absolute truths in the religious sense is a question of personal belief. Developmental studies cannot be used to support or refute this possibility, although they can show that knowledge of any such eternal realities cannot be innate nor inherited genetically.

This view that archetypes represent aspects of transcendental reality can apparently only be sustained by abandoning any attempt to consider them as biological entities, as some authors have argued we should (Pietikainen 1998). Archetypes might then be seen as culturally rather than biologically emergent forms, as symbolic forms which are repeated across a range of societies because the human experience of birth, life and death has so much in common, whatever the cultural context.

However, there is another framework which does succeed in uniting the transcendental with the biological in an innovative and original way, a framework based on mathematics. This view emerges in the writing of an analytical psychologist, Maxson McDowell (2001), a molecular biologist who, like Hogenson (2001) and Saunders and Skar (2001), rejects the idea that archetypes are hard-wired into the genes. However, he takes issue with their idea that archetypes are the emergent products of the self-organizing brain. Instead he draws on mathematical understanding to suggest that it is the inherent properties, which reliably determine the outcome of the process of self-organization, that are archetypal, rather than the products of that process.

McDowell has cogently argued that archetypes are mathematical principles or rules that govern psychological development, just as they govern the forms that emerge out of physical development. These mathematical principles are not inherited but are inherent in the processes that guide development. Mathematical rules reliably produce certain patterns in the inanimate world, such as whirlpools in turbulent water and in living forms, the repeated emergence of features such as wings across a range of different phyla and classes of animals.

It seems reasonable to suggest that mathematical rules may also govern the way in which the human mind categorizes and classifies information about the world. Mathematics is a form of abstract reality that exists independently of the biological world and could be considered to be a form of eternal truth, but one that, nevertheless, affects the functioning of the human mind.

However, a key question remains – what are the mental mechanisms whereby the human mind apprehends these mathematical principles and recognizes their applicability to the symbolic and emotional world? We have already found the answer to this question in the concept of the image schema. The mathematical rules that govern the world of physical objects are encapsulated in the image schema Gestalts that are formed as the very first stage of conceptual development and which I have described above. McDowell (2001) gives an example of complex imagery, fantasy and mythology that derives from the mathematical principle of splitting or division. 'Splitting' is one of the core image schemata that Johnson (1987) lists. In fact, because image schemata are formed from bodily experience of the physical world, they must represent the mathematical rules that govern physical movement and the relationships between objects in the physical world.

Conclusions

Archetypes are not in themselves innate, genetic structures. The evidence from developmental research suggests that archetypes can be equated with image schemas, the spatial models that are formed very early in the process of mental development and encode core information about the spatial relationships of objects in the world around us. These Gestalts then act as a base for extensive elaboration of these patterns into the symbolic world.

We may also be able to conclude that McDowell's model of the archetype as an inherent mathematical principle can be reconciled with the model of the archetype as image schema. The image schema embodies the abstract principle, representing it as a Gestalt stored in the human mind, available for further processing and extension into the world of imagination and metaphor.

The archetype is an emergent structure, derived from the self-organizing development of the human brain, as Saunders and Skar (2001) propose. Although I reject Saunders and Skar's proposal that archetypes are a form of complex, I do agree that archetypes are the early products of developmental self-organization. The image schema meets this requirement as it is the earliest representational structure that emerges from this process. This developmental model for archetypes requires us to recategorize them, removing them from the realm of innate mental content and acknowledging them as early products of mental development.

The earliest psychic structures, image schemas, offer a contemporary developmental model for archetypes, in that they organize experience while they themselves remain without content and beyond the realm of conscious awareness. The image schema would seem to correspond to the archetype-as-such and the archetypal image can be equated with the innumerable metaphorical extensions that derive from image schemas. McDowell's concept of the archetype as an inherent principle of psychic organization can be incorporated into this model, since each image schema embodies certain mathematical principles, expressing them as spatial, abstract dynamic patterns of relationship between objects.

Archetypes as psychic patterns of relationship rather than specific contents

The image schema model allows us to conclude that archetypes can contribute significantly to the internal object world. The metaphorical extensions of the image schema can provide a rich source of imagery and fantasy. However, the character of this imagery derives from the underlying image schema and image schemas are abstract organizing Gestalts of an impersonal nature. Thus, there may be no such thing as an archetypal mother but, instead, there is an image schema of containment.

A child's experience of his or her mother as physically and psychologically containing is a metaphorical extension of this image schema, or archetype-as-such. The Gestalt of containment is simple, but it can give rise to a wealth of meaning as it is expressed in the richness of physical intimacy and the mother's understanding and containment of her child's needs and emotions.

There would therefore seem to be an image-schematic or archetypal quality to almost any experience, and this developmental model of the image schema would thus seem to strengthen the concept of the archetype, enabling us to identify the key image-schematic features of an event, memory, dream or fantasy that justify us in using the term archetypal. The archetypal aspect of any experience lies in the pattern of relationship between the objects or people, a pattern that can be traced back to the underlying image

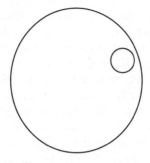

Figure 1   Diagram of containment

schema. 'Secure' parents provide an experience of safety and containment which is rooted in the image schema of 'containment' (Figure 1) and enablement (Johnson 1987: 126).

In contrast, intrusive parents who impose on their infant while failing to notice or respond to his or her communications are likely to activate the image schema of 'force' or 'splitting'.

In his investigation of the relationship between Jungian psychotherapy and contemporary infant research, Jacoby (1999) at times lends support to this model of the archetype as a process, referring to 'the archetypal organization of our experiences and behaviour' and to 'archetypal processes involved in the maturation of humans' (Jacoby 1999: 58). Unfortunately, Jacoby does not explore the possible contribution of the image schema to the concept of archetypes and does not mention the recent developmental research which increasingly underpins the self-organizing, emergent model of the human psyche. He also seems to preserve an allegiance to a concept of the archetype as a structure with specific representational content, for example, frequently referring to the mother archetype. I hope that I have clearly demonstrated the extent to which this content-orientated model of the archetype is incompatible with a contemporary developmental model of the human mind and have convinced the reader of the need to adopt a view of the archetype as a process and emergent pattern of relationship that provides meaning for the infant's perception of the physical world and of human relationships.

The image schema enables us to see clearly that it is the dynamic pattern of relationships of the objects of our inner world that is archetypal, rather than the specific characteristics of any particular object in inner or outer reality.

In Chapter 4 I want to investigate the way in which the principle of self-organization helps us to understand how unconscious meaning is constantly evolving and developing in the adult human mind and to relate this to Jung's concept of complexes and to some of the research findings from attachment theory.

I have highlighted the research evidence to show that, while complex symbolic meaning is never innate, it may be derived from metaphorical extension and elaboration of mental structures that are formed at a very early stage of the developmental process.

I shall now move on to explore the other, later developing, processes whereby unconscious meaning is constantly extracted from the kaleidoscope of our daily experience of the world. Archetypes, as image schemas that embody mathematical rules and have arisen out of the self-organizing development of the human brain, may play a key role in creating unconscious meaning, but they are not the only mechanisms by which the human mind orders experience. More complex symbolic and conceptual meaning depends on other cognitive processes which I shall investigate in Chapter 4. I shall explore the characteristics of internal objects and show that we need to move on to think of these as unconscious representations of dynamic patterns of relationship between self and other, in place of the traditional more static model which focuses on the specific representational content of the object. This new perspective will be seen to reflect the similar change in the concept of the archetype that I have explored in this chapter.

Chapter 4

The making of meaning

The formation of internal working models

In Chapter 3 I explored the evidence for the role that innate processes play in the development of human mental functioning, showing that genes trigger developmental processes, which then in their turn 'switch on' other genes, in a constant interactive sequence. In this chapter I want to change the focus of this inquiry away from the genetic and developmental processes that lie behind human mental functioning. I am now going to investigate the way the human mind interacts with the external world, how it processes experiences and events, stores information about them and then organizes that stored knowledge in a form that can be drawn on in order to make sense of further new experiences. This leads us to take a closer look at internal objects, the unconscious psychic structures which provide the substrate of our clinical analytic work.

A distinguishing hallmark of the analytic attitude is the focus on lasting psychic change within the patient, in contrast to a reliance on a change in behaviour which often characterizes other treatment modalities. The nature of this psychic change is a transformation in the patients' internal objects and in the pattern of relationships in their unconscious world, changes which can be identified through the transference–countertransference dynamics, and the pattern of unconscious meaning revealed in the narrative that unfolds in each analytic session.

The internal object thus seems to be a concept that unites analysts and psychotherapists from all theoretical schools. It performs this vital function because it is elastic enough to expand and to include the central tenets of each model of the psyche; for example, 'classical' psychoanalysts can integrate the Oedipus complex and the superego with the world of internal objects, while contemporary psychoanalysts can relate the internal object to the attachment theory concept of the 'internal working model'. For Kleinians, unconscious phantasy, splitting and projective identification form an integral part of object relations theory. More recently, contemporary analytical psychologists have extended our understanding of archetypes and complexes through an object relations approach. The internal object therefore seems to provide an indispensable service, giving us a language that we all understand and so allowing us to communicate with each other without losing the professional identities and loyalties each of us has acquired through immersion in the theory and practice of our respective trainings

The object relations model has, in fact, become something which is almost too precious to tamper with because all psychotherapists need it so much. It can be argued that this model constitutes the foundation stone of our theory and practice, in that our work with the unconscious world of internal objects is the characteristic that distinguishes psychodynamic therapy from all other psychological therapies. It may sometimes feel as though we question this world at our peril. Indeed, the Controversial Discussions in the British Psychoanalytic Society in the 1930s and 1940s demonstrate the profound disagreement and even hostility that can arise when analysts debate the nature of the internal object world among themselves.

On the other hand, since a central part of psychoanalytic work involves the most detailed exploration of the nature and functioning of our patients' internal objects, an investigation of this concept in the light of research in cognitive science and developmental psychology would help us establish the degree of scientific evidence in support of the models we use. However, such a study is fraught with difficulty because within both psychodynamic theory and cognitive science there are multiple definitions and theories concerning the nature of internal objects and the way they have arisen.

One of the questions which arises out of this diversity is whether cognitive science and psychodynamic theory refer to the same entities when describing the objects of the internal world. Greenberg and Mitchell (1983) argue that the objects of academic psychology are quite different from the objects of psychoanalysis, in that the former are simply entities existing in time and space, whereas in psychoanalysis the word 'object' sometimes refers to the target of a drive and sometimes to the internal images and residues of relations with real important people in an individual's life, which have been internalized and come to shape subsequent attitudes and perceptions (Greenberg and Mitchell 1983: 13). However, since the publication of Greenberg and Mitchell's work, a great deal more research has been done by cognitive scientists on the ways in which experiences and perceptions are taken in and stored in memory, leading to the formation of mental representations, the term used in cognitive science to describe information stored in the mind.

Internal objects can be thought of as a special category of mental representations. Marcel (1988) offers a clear summary of the concept of mental representations in cognitive science, a concept which does not seem significantly different from some psychoanalytic definitions of internal objects; he says that

> we happen to lead the lives we do lead, of a relatively organized kind, by reference to a representation of our environment, of our relation to it, of our past, and of our present moment-to-moment self-state. Without access to such representations we would be much more dependent on our immediate circumstances and much more rigid.
>
> (Marcel 1988: 141)

Although the content of mental representations has a different focus in psychodynamic theory and in cognitive science, in that psychodynamic theory is primarily about representations of people and of emotional relationships to the exclusion of representations of physical objects, this distinction is not always preserved. Marcel's definition provides a clear link between the concept of mental representation and that of the internal object.

I do not, therefore, think that Perlow (1995) draws valid conclusions in stating that psychoanalytic and cognitive science concepts of mental representations lie in vastly different domains and that psychoanalysis has little use for the format or process of representation, while cognitive science does not concern itself with the contents of representations in different individuals. The long-established concept of schemas proposed by Bartlett (1932) of 'an active organization of past reactions, or of past experiences, which must always be supposed to be operating in any well-adapted organic response' is a cognitive science model which does specify the content of schemas and clearly acknowledges the central role of the individual's unique experience in shaping mental representations (Bartlett 1932: 201; Perlow 1995: 151).

On the other side of the picture, psychodynamic theory does not concern itself solely with content, but has always drawn up complex models to explain the process of formation of representations, particularly in infancy. The focus on the forces that influence the formation of representations started with Freud who initially postulated that there is a progression through oral, anal and genital stages, each of which determines the focus of the infant's attention and so powerfully influences the nature of the mental representations formed (Freud 1905: 125–245). Melanie Klein (1932) developed the concept of part-objects and their integration in the depressive position into whole objects. She suggested that, in the early months of an infant's life, phantasies of an extreme polarized nature arise directly as a consequence of the operation of the 'life' and 'death' instincts (Klein 1932: 132).

Jung also offered ideas about the processes by which the mind organizes information; he formulated the idea of complexes which he described as unconscious structures with innate mental content. Fordham later developed Jung's ideas with the concept of the formation of mental representations through a cycle of deintegration, the activation of innate mechanisms, or archetypes, by an environmental stimulus, followed by reintegration, the formation of representations of the information, organized by the innate mechanism (Fordham 1985).

Johnson-Laird (1991) makes a point which goes to the heart of the issue in discussing the term 'mental model'. He points out that although mental models may differ markedly in their content, there is no evidence that they differ in representational format or in the processes that construct and manipulate them (Johnson-Laird 1991: 484). In that case, there is no reason to assume that mental representations of self–other relationships, which are the concern of psychodynamic theory, differ in format or formation from any other, even though their content is fairly specific and different from that of the mental representations which are usually the focus of study in cognitive science.

Peter Fonagy (2001) spells out the significance of Johnson-Laird's ideas for our understanding of the psyche, showing that we appraise the meaning of situations, not on the basis of formal rules of logic but instead on the basis of activation and manipulation of the particular mental model in operation. He writes:

Mental model theory assumes that to understand is to construct mental models from knowledge and from perceptual or
verbal evidence. To formulate a conclusion is to describe what
is represented in the models. To test validity is to search for
alternative models that refute the putative conclusion.

(Fonagy 2001: 120)

Fonagy goes on to suggest that mental model theory explains
irrationality and invalid deductions because these are emergent
features of mental models as they are constructed.

Object relations theory and its roots in drive theory: developmental considerations

Since the mid-1980s considerable excitement has been generated by
the work of developmental psychologists such as Daniel Stern
(1985), Wilma Bucci (1997) and Allan Schore (1994), who brought
neurobiological and developmental research to bear on psychoanalytic models of the mind and of its internal objects, research
which I shall discuss more fully later. However, Schore himself
points out that Freud's seminal treatise, 'Project for a scientific
psychology' (1895), was the earliest attempt to comprehensively
explain psychological phenomena in terms of neurobiological
explanatory models. The key features of this model were:

that the infant was relatively passive and undifferentiated, and
that its primary motivational aims were associated with
tension-discharging, drive-reducing activities. The infant's
awareness of objects was viewed as secondary to the fulfilment
of oral needs.

(Schore 1994: 24)

In Freud's mature psychoanalytic theory the instinctual drives,
specifically libido and the death instinct, are the direct source of
unconscious phantasy and hence the forces that determine the
content of internal objects. This approach is sustained in the full
flowering of the Kleinian object relations model and the root of
unconscious phantasy in instinctual drive was most clearly
expounded by Susan Isaacs (1948) in her article 'On the nature
and function of phantasy'. Hinshelwood (1989) points out how far
reaching this idea was, that:

all mental activity takes place on the basis of phantasied relations with objects, including the activity of perception, phantasied as a concrete incorporation through the perceptual apparatus, and thoughts as objects . . . unconscious phantasy, being the mental representation of instinctual impulses, is the nearest psychological phenomenon to the biological nature of the human being.

(Hinshelwood 1989: 34)

The primacy of unconscious phantasy as the focus for analytic work was highlighted by Joan Riviere, a strong supporter of Melanie Klein, when she wrote: 'Psychoanalysis is Freud's discovery of what goes on in the imagination . . . it has no concern with anything else, it is not concerned with the real world' (quoted in Rayner 1992). Joan Riviere was John Bowlby's analyst; his development of attachment theory, a model in which external reality plays a key part in the formation of the internal world, was partly a reaction against this position.

There is considerable research evidence which, though not definitive, does suggest that infants of the age of 6 months and under simply do not have the cognitive capacity for the kind of elaborate mental imagery which Klein proposed, which she considered to arise directly from instinctual drive (Stern 1985: 254–5). She described this as unconscious phantasy and thought, for example, that it included phantasies of the good and bad breast and of sadistic attacks on the mother's body. Klein (1952) wrote:

If we consider the picture which exists in the infant's mind – as we can see it retrospectively in the analyses of children and adults – we find that the hated breast has acquired the oral-destructive qualities of the infant's own impulses when he is in states of frustration and hatred. In his destructive phantasies he bites and tears up the breast, devours it, annihilates it; and he feels that the breast will attack him in the same way. As urethral- and anal-sadistic impulses gain in strength, the infant in his mind attacks the breast with poisonous urine and explosive faeces and therefore expects it to be poisonous and explosive towards him. The details of his sadistic phantasies determine the content of his fear of internal and external persecutors, primarily of the retaliating bad breast.

(Klein 1952: 63)

However, this kind of mental imagery would require the cognitive capacity to hold some kind of concept of the breast or other object in mind (even though such a concept may not be expressible in language) and also to attribute intentions to objects such as the breast. Accumulating research evidence suggests that infants of under 6 months do not have these cognitive capacities; such evidence has been extensively reviewed by Mandler (1988), Gergely (1992) and Beck (1998: 155). Two examples can illustrate the kind of research which does cast doubt on the developmental timetable of the Kleinian model of the infant mind.

Gergely *et al.* (1995) conducted visual habituation experiments which showed that the ability to attribute intentions to others does not emerge until the age of 12 months and that there are alternative explanations for previous empirical claims that this capacity emerges in the second half of the first year.

Second, as I discussed in Chapter 3, Jean Mandler argues that concept formation depends upon perceptual analysis 'a symbolic process . . . by which one perception is actively compared with another' (Mandler 1988: 126). She suggests that such comparisons involve categorization and that perceptual analysis always demonstrates that an analytic process is at work, doing conceptual thought rather than primitive recognition. She further argues that in the preverbal child perceptual analysis is the only route whereby information can become stored in an accessible representational system. Mandler (1988, 1992) cites a range of experiments, including those by Fox *et al.* (1979), which appeared to demonstrate that the active comparison of stimuli develops from about 6 months onwards, demonstrating that perceptual analysis begins to develop at that age (see the discussion of image schema formation in Chapter 4). The implication of these findings is that even the most primitive concept formation begins only at about 6 months, so that infants under this age would not have the cognitive capacities for concept formation that Kleinian theory requires. In addition, the earliest concepts formed from 6 months onwards are likely to be general categorizations of objects, for example into animate or inanimate, without detailed featural analysis (Mandler 1992: 590–1). Concepts such as 'breast', 'urine' or 'faeces' would seem to be too detailed and specific for the developing cognitive capacities of the 3–6 month old, according to the model offered by Mandler.

The view that instinctual drives are the major determinant of the nature of internal objects was first seriously challenged by Fairbairn

(1941), who proposed that the infant's behaviour is primarily relationship-seeking from the start and that it is impossible to understand psychic functioning out of the context of early relationships. Guntrip, Balint and others of the British Object Relations school shared this view and Anna-Ursula Dreher describes the steady move in psychoanalysis away from drive theory, as:

> the gradual transition in psychoanalytic thought from a model of economics and dynamics of *drives* and energies, of drive discharge and restraining structures, towards a model of the economics and dynamics of *feeling states*, reflecting the full range from anxiety, depression, and pain to well-being and safety.
>
> (Dreher 2000: 109, original emphases)

Dreher goes on to highlight the

> gradual but clear transformation of mainstream psychoanalysis from a psychology of the drives into a mature object-relations perspective, which today is generally regarded as the perspective of the 'contemporary Freudians'. It focuses on self and object representations and on experiences of interactions and feeling states, both of which have sedimented within these representations and, in turn, this perspective leads to the differentiation of the concept of the ego as the executive agent of adaptation and regulation of such feeling states.
>
> (Dreher 2000: 109)

Joseph Sandler and other representational theorists also favour this model of internal objects as representation or schemas

> an amalgamation of all experiences the individual has of his objects, including his actual interactions with them and their emotional meanings, as well as the distortions of realistic aspects under influences of drives and phantasies. As such, a mental representation of an object refers to a schema, which on the basis of past experience (not necessarily realistic) organizes present experience and provides a context for both present perceptions and for the recall of past memories.
>
> (Perlow 1995: 149–50)

This is very different from the Kleinian model which I outlined earlier.

This model of internal objects as representations, formed in large part from the internalization of external experiences and 'experienced' in the form of a guide, is increasingly accepted by many contemporary Freudian and Jungian analysts (Eagle 1995; Knox 1999). Developmental psychology research is calling into question the validity of drive theory, while the key role of representations of real experience in the formation of mental representations has support from experimental research (Emde 1992; Stern 1994). Research by Stern (1994), Lichtenberg (1981) and Bucci (1997) among others has demonstrated the cognitive capacities of early infancy and offers us a contemporary model of the human psyche. From birth, the human infant is exploring the world, seeking and responding to crucial stimuli in the environment, integrating information gained from different modalities and relating to these experiences as a whole person with whole objects, even though this relationship is initially sensation-based and operates at a primitive cognitive level.

From object relations to attachment theory

The British Object Relations school may be thought of as a precursor of attachment theory but it lacks some of the key features which Bowlby (1969, 1973) introduced into his fully developed model of attachment theory. He became increasingly uneasy with the emphasis of psychoanalytic theory on autonomous intrapsychic processes which seemed to him to neglect the role of interpersonal relationships in the formation of the internal world. He became particularly critical of the Kleinian model, which placed instinctual drive theory at the heart of psychoanalysis. Bowlby felt that this was a view which seemed to render the environment virtually insignificant in its contribution to the formation of psychic contents. On the other hand, attachment theory may, at first sight, seem to have something in common with conditioning or behavioural models in the sense that environmental influences play a key role. The critical point of attachment theory is that cumulative experiences are internalized to form unconscious 'internal working models' which guide expectations and perceptions, so serving as a template for future relationships.

In fact, one of the most significant innovations that Bowlby introduced was his replacement of the concept of the internal object with that of the internal working model, which offers a more accurate description, in cognitive science terms, of the way information is processed and stored implicitly than the term 'internal object'. Bowlby described internal working models in some detail:

> Starting, we may suppose, towards the end of his first year, and probably especially active during his second and third when he acquires the powerful and extraordinary gift of language, a child is busy constructing working models of how the physical world might be expected to behave, how his mother and other significant persons might be expected to behave, how he himself might be expected to behave, and how each interacts with the other. Within the framework of these working models he evaluates his situation and makes his plans. And within the framework of these working models of his mother and himself he evaluates special aspects of his situation and makes his attachment plans.
>
> (Bowlby 1969: 354)

Internal working models contain complex representational information about patterns of relationship, particularly of self in relation to key attachment figures. Bowlby apparently preferred the term 'internal working model' to that of 'map' or 'image' because it conveys the sense that the pattern contained in the model can be drawn on to predict events and behaviour (Bretherton and Munholland 1999: 91). Indeed, the internal working model can be considered as the theoretical foundation stone of attachment theory in that it describes the infant's capacity for holding his or her mother (and others) in mind when she is not present. Internal working models can exist only in infants' minds when they are capable of representation, of forming a working model of their mother which is available to them for the purposes of comparison during her absence and for recognition after her return.

Bowlby was also quite clear that instinctual drives play no part in the formation of the internal world and that unconscious phantasy is not an expression of libido or the death instinct (Bowlby 1988: 70). Although Bowlby was in analysis with Melanie Klein and later with Joan Riviere, he completely rejected his Kleinian heritage, describing Klein as 'totally unaware of the scientific method'

(Fonagy 1999b: 605). For Bowlby and for subsequent attachment theorists, an unbridgeable gulf exists between the psychoanalytic model in which instinctual drives give rise to unconscious phantasy and largely define the nature of internal objects, and an attachment theory view of the psyche, in which internal working models are gradually constructed from the wealth of accumulated experience of the real world and of actual relationships with key attachment figures. Peter Fonagy points out that, although post-Kleinian psychoanalysts are more able to accept the role of the environment in shaping internal objects, 'at present there is no room in attachment theory for a concept such as the death instinct. Kleinian ideas continue to pivot around the innate destructiveness of the human infant' (Fonagy 2001: 91). Kernberg, for example, still regards instinctual drives as a major determinant of the content of 'internal objects' even though he describes them as self–object–affect triads (Kernberg 1988). Although contemporary psychoanalysts are moving towards an attachment-based model of the formation of unconscious psychic structures, some still regard instinctual drives as playing a significant role.

The meaning of internalization

Attachment theory therefore provides an alternative explanation to that of drive theory for the formation of internal objects; it is a model in which interpersonal experiences with key attachment figures are 'internalized' (encoded and stored as mental representations) and cumulative experiences of this kind are gradually built up in the mind into schematic representations of generalized patterns of such interactions called 'internal working models' (Bowlby 1988: 129). These internal working models influence a person's perceptions of, and attitudes and behaviour towards, all subsequent emotionally important relationships, but are not themselves accessible to conscious awareness. They therefore offer an account which is compatible with the experimental evidence for implicit memory and would seem to be a particular manifestation of its functioning with regard to the storage and retrieval of information of important relationships (Fonagy 1999a).

If attachment theory suggests that internalization is the key process underpinning the formation of internal objects, then we need to be clear exactly what the term means. In information-processing terms, internalization does not mean that some psychological material actually passes from one person to another, although it often seems to be used in a way that suggests this; even the term 'internal object' rather carries the connotation that some foreign body has been incorporated into one person's psyche from another's. Internalization is a description of the consequences of interpersonal experiences, but it is also an account of the information processing which goes on within one person's mind as a result of that two-person interaction.

This schematized record of interpersonal experiences offers an attachment theory account of internalization and distinguishes it from Bion's (1959) model, which suggests that mother and infant experience communication as though psychological material somehow passes between them. Bion describes this as an experience where thoughts and feelings are inserted from one to the other to explain the way that communicator and recipient might feel, but he does not provide an information-processing account to explain this experience (Bion 1959). Hinshelwood (1989) summarizes this as a process in which the

> mother's mind needs to be in a state of calm receptiveness to take in the infant's own feelings and give them meaning. The idea is that the infant will, through projective identification, insert into the mother's mind a state of anxiety and terror which he is unable to make sense of and which is felt to be intolerable.
>
> (Hinshelwood 1989: 404)

The maternal reverie makes sense of the infant's mental state and the infant takes this back inside (introjects) and so develops a capacity to reflect on his or her own states of mind.

In contrast, an attachment theory account of internal working models and patterns of attachment is a description of the information processing, within one person's mind, of interpersonal experience, and so does provide a more precise model for the experience of internalization.

Attachment theory as a bridge between psychodynamic theory and cognitive science

Attachment theory therefore can act as a bridge between psychodynamic theory and cognitive science because it offers a model of the psyche which is both dynamic and dependent on processes that are in keeping with current knowledge about the ways in which the mind encodes and stores information in memory. Grossman (1995) emphasizes the urgency of this bridge-building task, saying 'two psychologies have existed side by side for more than a hundred years, and the shakiness of the bridges between them has ever so often been deplored'. He goes on to state:

> Attachment is not one relationship among others; it is the very foundation of healthy individual development. More, it is the precondition for developing a coherent mind, even if it is, finally, insufficient by itself for understanding the whole mind. Scientifically, attachment theory has done nothing less than bridge the gap between individual experience and objective research.
>
> (Grossman 1995: 116)

For example, the concept of 'internal working models' gives an information-processing account of the way in which mental representations of relationships with key attachment figures are formed and stored in implicit memory, an account which is much more compatible with evidence from developmental psychology and research on the nature of memory than the psychodynamic concept of 'internal objects', as Bowlby himself suggested (Bowlby 1988: 120). As a further bridge to cognitive science, the retrieval of internal working models can be linked to the phenomena of state-dependent retrieval (in which any information learnt in one situation is preferentially recalled when a person is again in that situation) and of mood-congruent retrieval (in which an emotional state leads to preferential recall of information with the same emotional content). Relationships which retrieve a particular internal working model will also retrieve information learnt on previous occasions when that working model was retrieved, and the emotions which accompany the retrieved internal working model will lead to preferential recall of similar emotional experiences. This model successfully accounts, not only for the way we establish secure and loving relationships, but also for the repetition of maladaptive and destructive patterns of relationship which therapists so often see in their patients. An important motivational factor in the perpetuation of attachment patterns is the desire to reproduce a familiar relationship pattern, however destructive, precisely because it is familiar and understood. Adults unconsciously seek out relationships with people who replicate the patterns of early childhood experience, however unsatisfactory that may have been.

A key feature of attachment theory, which enables it to act as a conceptual bridge, is that it is a memory model which gives an account of the ways experiences of key relationships are registered and then organized and stored in memory. The central features of this memory model are:

- experience of real relationships is 'internalized';
- the representations of these relationships are stored as schemas, or working models and 'the form these models take is in fact far more strongly determined by a child's actual experiences throughout childhood than was formerly supposed';
- whatever representational models of attachment figures and of self an individual builds during his childhood and adolescence, these tend to persist into and throughout adult life;
- as a result, any new person to whom an attachment is formed becomes assimilated into an existing model and perceptions of that person are organized by the existing model, even in the face of evidence that the model is inappropriate;
- the influence that existing working models have on current perceptions operates outside awareness;
- inappropriate but persistent representational models often co-exist with more appropriate ones;
- the stronger the emotions aroused in a relationship the more likely are the earlier and less conscious models to become dominant.

(Bowlby 1979: 117 and 141)

For example, young children, about 5 years old, will have mental representations of their mother, containing olfactory, tactile, visual and verbal information about her physical presence, information about the physical, emotional and cognitive interactions between them and information about their own emotional responses to her presence and absence. At this age, children's representations of their mother will also contain some information about her relationship with their father, as well as with any siblings and others outside the family, such as their teachers and the mothers of other children. These representations are derived directly from these personal experiences. All this information is stored in the form of generalized 'rules' about mother, expectations or anticipatory sets about what sort of things she does and how she relates to her child; these are internal working models. For a securely attached child, the changing ways in which the parents treat him or her result in a gradual updating of these models; however, for an anxiously attached child, this gradual updating of models is obstructed by anxious avoidance of new patterns, so that early models persist even when the individual in later life is dealing with people who treat him/her entirely differently from the ways his/her parents treated him/her as a child (Bowlby 1988: 131).

Stern (1985) supports Bowlby's account with his own description of 'Representations of Interactions that have been Generalized', or RIGs, which are abstract representations, based on multiple specific memories and which form the basis for expectations about the likely course of events, actions, feelings and sensations in given situations (Stern 1985: 97). These abstract representations are of generalized episodes which are not specific memories of actual events, but are formed from multiple such specific memories from which generalized information is drawn. Internal working models therefore contain a vast range of generalized information about the external world and the subjective psychological state. They reflect the functioning of implicit memory and the fact that it is the relationship between self and other, as well the emotions which reflect that relationship, which are represented in memory.

Internal working models which contain generalized information about attachment figures and relationships, exist separately from memories containing explicit and conscious information about specific episodes in the relationship, perhaps about an exciting holiday, or the first time the child learnt to swim with the mother's help, or the time she took the child to the doctor to have a vaccination. Children's explicit, conscious memories of their mother will be stored as information of particular episodes, but they will also have information in implicit format in internal working models.

Transgenerational transmission of attachment patterns

Another key feature of internal working models is that they can be unconsciously communicated by a parent and internalized by the child. As Fraiberg and colleagues so evocatively said, 'in every nursery there are ghosts. These are the visitors from the unremembered pasts of the parents, the uninvited guests at the christening' (Fraiberg *et al.* 1975: 387–8). How do the parental ghosts become incorporated into the internal working models of the infant? The most striking evidence comes from studies which demonstrate that a parent's internal model of attachment as measured in the Adult Attachment Interview correlates with the child's security of attachment as measured by the Strange Situation. This shows that it is the parent's internal world which is the formative influence affecting the child's pattern of attachment.

It seems that parents' internal working models are communicated to and internalized by their children, becoming part of that child's internal world, in other words, part of that child's fantasy. There is considerable research evidence that demonstrates this kind of intergenerational transmission of attachment patterns and, by implication, the internal working models which underpin that behaviour. An experiment by Broussard (1970) explored mothers' fantasies about their babies soon after birth; they were asked to rate their first-born babies as better than average or not better than average at the end of the babies' first month. Babies whose mothers had rated them as 'not better than average' were three times more likely to show clinical psychological problems at the age of 4 than the babies whose mothers had rated them better than average at 1 month. The predictive power of the mother's initial fantasy of the worth of their infants continued to the age of 10 when the negatively viewed infants still had markedly greater diagnosable mental disorder than the more positively viewed babies.

Another key attachment theorist, Alicia Lieberman, has also explored the processes by which babies 'become the carriers of the parents' unconscious fears, impulses, and other repressed or disowned parts of themselves' and how these 'negative attributions become an integral part of the child's sense of self' (Lieberman 1999: 373). Parental projective identification has a profound impact on children, who are under great pressure to comply with the parents' need for them to act as repositories for the parents' intolerable emotions and states of mind and eventually enacts the role they have been assigned. It seems that children are vulnerable to this kind of pressure because they need to be loved by the parents even if the price is the development of a distorted sense of self as a result of parental projections, although Lieberman (1999) does not spell this out. The defensive aspects of the child's response to parental attributions will be explored in Chapter 5.

The characteristics of implicit memory

Fonagy (1999a) has expanded on the work of authors such as Clyman (1991) to suggest that implicit memory is the form in which generalized patterns of experiences are stored non-consciously, determining expectations of current events and relationships, but remaining outside awareness themselves (Clyman 1991; Fonagy 1999a).

Cognitive research provides evidence that recent experiences can influence performance and behaviour in the absence of conscious recollection of those experiences. This would allow for cognitive formation and processing of mental representations as a process separate, or dissociated, from conscious awareness. For example, Churchland (1988) presents evidence which demonstrates information processing without conscious awareness. She quotes research which showed that when women were asked to choose from identical items of clothing on a table they explained their choice in terms of colour, texture, etc. when in fact there was no difference in any of these factors and the only determining factor was that they chose items lying to the right-hand side of the table, but with no awareness that this determined their choice (Churchland 1988: 289).

There are also the experiments by Weiskrantz on blind sight and hemineglect. Weiskrantz (1986) found that subjects with hemianopia caused by unilateral damage to the striate cortex would, when asked, state that they did not see events in their 'blind' fields, but forced-choice methods showed that they have in fact accurately detected these events. Marcel's work on visual masking in normal subjects showed that perception occurred without conscious awareness (Marcel 1983). These research findings, whether of the kind occurring in normal subjects or characteristic of certain kinds of neurological damage, demonstrate that information processing goes on independently and outside of conscious awareness.

Schacter (1996) has extended the investigation of dissociation of conscious from non-conscious processing beyond the question of perceptual priming, showing that complex conceptual and semantic knowledge can be processed without conscious awareness (Schacter 1996: 189). He has used the term 'implicit memory' for

the kind of processing in which memory for conceptual information can be demonstrated on testing without any conscious recollection by the subject of that information. A most dramatic
example is given in an investigation of patients who have been
anaesthetized; it shows that they may process auditory information
during adequate anaesthesia; the presence of implicit memory for
events which occurred during anaesthesia is shown by a change in
test performance, attributable to information acquired, but without
having direct recollection of the event (Sebel 1995).

Unfortunately, the term 'implicit memory' is used with a variety
of meanings by different authors, with the terms 'implicit' and
'unconscious' sometimes used interchangeably even by writers
such as Schacter (1996), who sometimes refers to perceptual priming as a manifestation of implicit memory rather than reserving the
term for the storage of conceptual and semantic information in a
format which is inaccessible to consciousness. Perceptual priming
effects could be a manifestation of short-term storage in the 'visuo-
spatial sketch pad' of working memory, where information can be
held for very brief periods (Baddeley and Hitch 1974); they may
not relate to any processing in long-term memory, either explicit or
implicit.

Since information in implicit memory is stored in the form of
abstract generalized patterns rather than as specific records of
particular events, this information is not available to conscious
recall. Internal working models can be activated and then influence
us outside of our conscious awareness. This will be discussed
further in relation to Jung's concept of the complex, which he
described in similar terms.

A key point I want to make here is that implicit memory stores
information about similarities of experience and thus offers an
account of the way in which unconscious core meanings emerge,
through the process of the internalization of experience and its
subsequent organization into generalized patterns in implicit
memory. It is by means of this process that unconscious 'core'
meanings emerge, rather than through the activation of some innate
predetermined pattern of meaning, the third model of the archetype
that I discussed in Chapters 2 and 3. The archetype, as image
schema, can certainly contribute to the underlying 'scaffolding' of
the core pattern of meaning (see discussion on pp. 55–7) but the
process of internalization and the abstract format of information
storage in implicit memory play the major role.

Analytical psychology and internal working models

At first sight it would seem as though analytical psychologists might have less trouble than psychoanalysts in integrating new perspectives on internal objects into our conceptual frameworks, in that Jung emphatically rejected instinctual drive as the source of unconscious fantasy. He wrote:

> Unlike Freud, who after a proper psychological start reverted to the ancient assumption of the sovereignty of the physical constitution, trying to turn everything back in theory into instinctual processes conditioned by the body, I start with the sovereignty of the psyche.
>
> (Jung 1921: para. 968)

Jung stated his rejection of sexuality as the source of psychic life quite clearly when he wrote: 'I cannot see the real aetiology of neurosis in the various manifestations of infantile sexual development and the fantasies to which they give rise' (Jung 1916: para. 574). This was one of the fundamental differences that finally brought about the permanent fracture of his relationship with Freud.

Although Jung fully acknowledged the crucial role that personal experience plays in the formation of the unconscious internal world he struggled in his attempt to provide an integrated account of the interaction of real experience with innate psychic content and he did not offer any significant discussion of psychological development in infancy and childhood. It was Michael Fordham who extended Jungian theory to the study of childhood development, drawing on psychoanalytic models to understand the formation of internal objects in infancy (Fordham 1969).

The Kleinian model of the formation of internal objects (outlined earlier) is one which has had considerable influence not only in psychoanalytic theory but also on the models of developmentally orientated Jungians. This does create certain theoretical incompatibilities which Jungians have not really addressed because Jung himself emphatically rejected Freud's instinctual drive theory, arguing that the innate structures of the human mind do not come with prepackaged mental contents, but instead are predispositions which organize information coming from the environment. However, the fact that there are certain similarities between his concept of archetypal polarization and the good and bad polarization of the Kleinian model is not enough to overcome the fundamental differences between the two theoretical frameworks. In Klein's model of phantasy, the contents of the phantasy arise from within as though certain images pre-exist fully formed in the brain and are waiting to be released by a good feed or an experience of frustration. Although Klein acknowledged the role of external reality in contributing to unconscious phantasy, it only seems to play the part of a trigger which releases innate unconscious phantasies. Jung on the contrary understood that mental imagery always has its origin in external experience, which is then internalized and modified by archetypal expectation, a position considerably expanded and amplified by Fordham.

The concept of the 'complex'

The theory of the complex was introduced by Jung during the early stages of his collaboration with Freud, who was also initially enthusiastic about the concept but later rejected it when his final break with Jung occurred in 1913. I have previously outlined the similarities between Jung's model of the complex and the concept of the 'internal working model' offered by attachment theory (Knox 1999) and I will now review this similarity more fully.

Jung's concept of the complex is rooted in that of dissociation which, in turn, is related to Janet's (1925[1919]) formulation of the concept, as Ellenberger (1970) highlights:

> C.G. Jung repeatedly referred to Janet (whose lectures he had attended in Paris during the winter semester (1902–1903)). The influence of *Psychological Automatism* can be seen from Jung's way of considering the human mind as comprising a number of sub-personalities (Janet's 'simultaneous psychological existences'). What Jung called 'complex' was originally nothing but the equivalent of Janet's 'subconscious fixed idea'.
>
> (Ellenberger 1970: 406)

Emotion is included in the functioning of these dissociated parts of the mind called 'complexes'. Jung was clear that the 'feeling-tone', or emotion, holds clusters of memories together in an unconscious grouping which is dissociated from the rest of mental functioning; these clusters of emotionally based representations exist as a normal phenomenon as well as contributing to psychopathology. This seems to me to be fairly close to a model of complexes as schemas, partly conscious and partly unconscious patterns which organize perception and memory.

Roger Brooke in *Jung and Phenomenology* underlines the point that, for Jung, the unconscious is a dissociated rather than a dynamically repressed unconscious (Brooke 1991: 126). In the classical Jungian position, 'the unconscious' is conceived as an autonomous structure. Dissociation gives rise to complexes which are fragmentary personalities or splinter psyches and the ego is only one complex among many. Within these complexes, there is perception, feeling, volition and intention, as though a subject were present which thinks and is goal-directed. The unconscious is thus multiple consciousnesses. Consciousness is a consequence of the ego's capacity to appropriate as one's own and use effectively and freely the complexes that are already structuring one's existence. Without the ego's self-reflection, the complexes function automatically and have a compulsive quality.

One of the best summaries of Jung's concept of dissociation and its contribution to the formation of complexes is given by Sandner and Beebe:

> Jung thought that whatever its roots in previous experience, neurosis consists of a refusal – or inability- in the here and now to bear legitimate suffering. Instead this painful feeling or some representation of it is split off from awareness and the initial wholeness – the primordial Self – is broken. Such splitting 'ultimately derives from the apparent impossibility of affirming the whole of one's nature' (Jung 1934: 980) and gives rise to the whole range of dissociations and conflicts characteristic of feeling-toned complexes. This splitting is a normal part of life. Initial wholeness is meant to be broken, and it becomes pathological, or diagnosable as illness, only when the splitting off of complexes becomes too wide and deep and the conflict too intense. Then the painful symptoms may lead to the conflicts of neurosis or to the shattered ego of psychosis.
>
> (Sandner and Beebe 1984: 296)

They point out that complexes are living units,

> each carrying a splinter of consciousness of its own, a degree of
> intentionality, and the capability of pursuing a goal. They are
> like real personalities in that they contain images, feelings, and
> qualities and if they engulf the ego they determine behaviour as
> well.
>
> (Sandner and Beebe 1984: 298)

Jung's concept of the complex was also underpinned by his sound
empirical work on word association tests, which I will briefly
describe. Subjects are tested on 100 stimulus words, having been
instructed to react with the first word that comes into their mind as
quickly as possible after having heard and understood the stimulus
word; the reaction time to each stimulus word is measured with a
stop-watch and when the 100 words have been presented, they are
then re-presented, again one at a time, and the subjects have to
attempt to reproduce their former answers. In certain cases their
memory fails and reproduction becomes uncertain or faulty; Jung
concluded that these failures or delays in recall had 'hit on what I
call a complex, a conglomeration of psychic contents characterized
by a peculiar or perhaps painful feeling-tone, something that is
usually hidden from sight' (Jung 1935: paras. 97–106).

Jung gives striking clinical examples of the apparent effectiveness
of the word association test, one of which involved an apparently
'normal' subject, a man of 35, who produced abnormal reactions to
the words 'knife', 'lance', 'beat', 'pointed' and 'bottle'. After com-
pleting the test, Jung said, 'I did not know you had had such a
disagreeable experience', to which the man responded with 'I don't
know what you are talking about'. Jung stated that the man had
had a drunken quarrel and had stuck a knife into someone, which
the subject then acknowledged to be true.

Jung concluded from this kind of work that a complex
consisted of

> the *image* of a certain psychic situation which is strongly
> accentuated emotionally and is, moreover incompatible with
> the habitual attitude of consciousness. This image has a
> powerful inner coherence, it has its own wholeness and, in
> addition, a relatively high degree of autonomy, so that it is

subject to the control of the conscious mind only to a limited extent and therefore behaves like an animated foreign body in the sphere of consciousness.

(Jung 1934: paras. 200–3, original emphasis)

In this passage, Jung also emphasized that the existence of complexes throws

serious doubt on the naïve assumption of the unity of consciousness, which is equated with psyche, and on the supremacy of the will. Every constellation of a complex postulates a disturbed state of consciousness. The unity of consciousness is disrupted and the intentions of the will are impeded or made impossible. Even memory is often noticeably affected, as we have seen.

(Jung 1934: paras. 200–3)

Jung constantly emphasized the emotional basis of the complex and he also made it clear in the passage I have just quoted that he considered the contents of the complex to be mental representations, in this case taking the form of images.

Jung also recognized that emotion is not merely a visceral or physiological experience, but is inextricably bound up with cognition, a view which has been independently elaborated within an information-processing framework by George Mandler (1975: 47). Once again this differs from the Freudian view that instinctual drives are the root source of emotion.

Clinical illustration

A clinical example might best illustrate the models I have just described:

A female patient with bulimia has had several weeks in which she has maintained very good control of her eating and has felt emotionally stable without any of the bouts of severe distress and panic which usually lead her to binge. However my return from holiday seems to have immediately activated the severe distress, anxiety and desire to binge. She herself worked out that while I was away she was able to remain stable by holding an image of me as a benign and supportive parent figure in her mind, an image which was predictable and safe and under her control. On my return, she had to start relating to me as a real person again. The sense of the other person as separate and unpredictable makes her feel terrified that at any moment she will fail to meet that person's demands and that she has failed them. This emotional content acts as a cue which retrieves numerous implicit beliefs that she has failed, that the person she is trying to please will be angry with her and reject her; the content of these beliefs lacks any 'as-if' quality, so that she really believes that I might at any moment actually hit her in a session. These are both imaginative constructions of what she fears and memories of the many occasions on which her parents hit her if she did something to displease them.

Thus, the emotional experience of dependence on people who are powerful and whom she cannot control activates implicit beliefs about herself as a failure and as the object of hostility and rejection; these beliefs form a complex, dissociated from consciousness when she is on her own, but which takes over and dominates her awareness when she is in close contact with people who are important to her.

She has known this for some time without that insight producing any noticeable change in this pattern of relationships; however we have both recently recognized that there is another level of assumptions and beliefs which had until now remained unconscious. It has become apparent that whenever she feels that she has failed or might fail, she fears rejection not only for what she has done, but also for being the person who has done those things; she feels annihilated as a person, that she is totally bad, disgusting and unlovable and would be better off dead. The sense of failure in relation to something she has done activates negative beliefs about her very identity, a sense of failure for being the person she is. It is apparently the activation of these beliefs which triggers her bingeing, an activity which I have interpreted as a desperate attempt to treat herself as mindless and so without an identity which could be destroyed by rejection in the way she has so often experienced.

The anxiety generated by the activated complexes, which make her feel that she is totally unlovable and of no value, is so intolerable that there is an intentional imaginative creation of representations of herself as mindless, with only bodily needs. Thus there is a kind of 'cascade', starting with the anxiety about being with people, which activates a sense of failure and of being the object of criticism and hostility; these then retrieve other internal working models of herself as disgusting and unlovable and these in turn retrieve models containing representations of herself as mindless, representations which are linked to a compulsion to binge and which can be described as 'defensive' because they allow her to avoid paying attention to the representations of herself as disgusting and unlovable.

These ideas and images could all be seen as forming the content of a complex, which is dissociated from her consciousness when she is alone and feels emotionally safe, but which is activated by the emotional experience of dependence and the anxiety that accompanies this.

Many of these ideas are strikingly compatible with the findings of contemporary research-based cognitive science in a way in which many original Freudian and Kleinian theoretical formulations, such as 'drives', the 'death instinct' and 'unconscious phantasy' are not. Jung regards psychic contents as mental representations, images formed in a large part from actual childhood experience rather than generated by unconscious phantasy:

> More and more the neurologist of today realizes that the origin of the nervousness of his patients is very rarely of recent date but goes back to the early impressions and developments in childhood.
>
> (Jung 1919: para. 1793)

Perhaps even more striking is his recognition of the unconscious nature of the parent's influence on the child, a key feature of the intergenerational transmission of attachment patterns. Jung wrote:

> Parents too easily content themselves with the belief that a thing hidden from the child cannot influence it. They forget that infantile imitation is less concerned with action than with the parent's state of mind from which the action emanates. I have frequently observed children who were particularly influenced by certain unconscious tendencies in the parents and, in

such cases, I have often advised the treatment of the mother rather than of the child.

(Jung 1919: para. 1793)

This remark is strikingly similar to Fraiberg *et al.*'s (1975) comment that there are ghosts from the unremembered past of the parents in every nursery.

Jung's description of the dissociated nature of consciousness, his awareness of the crucial part played by internalization and inter-generational transmission in the formation of unconscious contents have much in common with the contemporary view of cognitive scientists.

The contribution of the archetype/image schema to the formation of internal objects

Although Jung developed an account of the relationship between external reality and the mental representations which form the content of the 'complex', he also thought that the complex was organized around an innate core. He said that the complex is 'embedded' in the material of the personal unconscious, but that its 'nucleus' consists of an archetypal core, archetypes being 'systems of readiness for action, and at the same time images and emotions'. Complexes are 'feeling-toned groups of representations' in the unconscious and consist of 'innate' (archetypal) patterns of expectation combined with external events which are internalized and given meaning by the 'innate' pattern (Jacobi 1959: 6). This leads me to investigate a contemporary way of describing the role of the archetype in the formation of the complex by identifying it with the contribution of the image schema to the internal working model.

In Chapter 3, I described the evidence from developmental research which demonstrates the existence of Gestalt-type mental structures which are probably the earliest products emerging from the self-organization of the human brain, a process that continues from birth and probably starts even *in utero* (Piontelli 1992). This developmental model for archetypes requires us to recategorize them, removing them from the realm of innate mental content and acknowledging them as early products of mental development. In this way, analytical psychologists can avoid falling into the same trap as psychoanalysts who regard instinctual drives as the main source of unconscious phantasy. Any suggestion that the human mind contains innate preformed packets of imagery and phantasy, waiting to pop out given the right environmental trigger, is outdated and to be discredited.

However, image schemas, early developmental mental structures which organize experience while themselves remaining without content and beyond the realm of conscious awareness, offer a contemporary developmental model for archetypes. The image schema would seem to correspond to the archetype-as-such, and the archetypal image can be equated with the innumerable metaphorical extensions that derive from image schemas. McDowell's (2001) concept of the archetype as an inherent principle of psychic organization can be incorporated into this model, since each image schema embodies certain mathematical principles, expressing them as spatial, abstract dynamic patterns of relationship between objects.

It would therefore be logical to conclude that archetypes can contribute significantly to the internal object world. The metaphorical extensions of the image schema can provide a rich source of imagery and fantasy. However, the character of this imagery derives from the underlying image schema and image schemas are abstract organizing Gestalts of an impersonal nature. Thus, there may be no such thing as an archetypal mother but, instead, there is an image schema of containment.

A child's experience of the mother as physically and psychologically containing is a metaphorical extension of this image schema, or archetype-as-such. The Gestalt of containment is simple but it can give rise to a wealth of meaning as it is expressed in the richness of physical intimacy and the parent's understanding and containment of her child's needs and emotions.

There would therefore seem to be an image-schematic or archetypal quality to almost any experience and this developmental model of the image schema would thus seem to strengthen the concept of the archetype but at the same time to identify the key features of an event, memory, dream or fantasy that justify us in using the term archetypal. I would remind the reader of the conclusion that I drew at the end of Chapter 3 that:

> The image schema enables us to see clearly that it is the dynamic pattern of relationships of the objects of our inner world that is archetypal, rather than the specific characteristics of any particular object in inner or outer reality.

Neurobiological perspectives on the nature of internal objects

Since the early 1980s, research evidence has begun to accumulate which demonstrates that early attachment relationships and experiences have a significant impact on the neurological development of the human brain in various ways. To give two brief examples, Schore has described in extraordinary detail the evidence that demonstrates that 'neurodevelopmental processes of dendritic proliferation and synaptogenesis which are responsible for postnatal brain growth are critically influenced by events at interpersonal and intrapersonal levels' (Schore 1994: 160). LeDoux has also described the physiological mechanisms whereby learning involves the strengthening of synaptic connections between neurones (LeDoux 1998: 213). Can neurobiological evidence tell us about the mechanisms in the brain that are responsive to the environment and about the processes that are called into play as day-to-day experiences are evaluated and stored in memory, some as explicit memories that can be consciously recalled and some as unconscious patterns in implicit memory? What are the neurological mechanisms that underpin the formation of internal working models? What factors determine the nature of information which is included in memory and, perhaps even more importantly, that which is excluded?

Bowlby himself was aware of the need to provide an information-processing account of the formation of internal working models:

> Sensory inflow goes through many stages of selection, interpretation and appraisal before it can have any influence on behaviour, either immediately or later. This processing occurs in a succession of stages, all but the preliminary of which require that the inflow be related to matching information already stored in long-term memory.
>
> (Bowlby 1980: 45)

The key issue is that there is not a simple one-stage process for inclusion or exclusion of information in memory. As Cortina points out, viewing the processing of information in general and defensive processes in particular, as operating in multiple stages that are coordinated with memory systems, offers a new paradigm for understanding the way the mind works. He writes: 'Appraising, selecting and interpreting experience is not a function of an agency of the mind such as the id or the ego or superego; *it is what the brain does*' (Cortina 2003, original emphasis). Cortina goes on to link the processes by which the mind selects, sorts and stores information with Edelman's view of the neurological mechanisms which underpin them:

> According to Edelman the brain is perpetually in the process of recreating itself through two twin processes: neuronal group selection and re-entrant signalling. We constantly confront new information and new situations. How does the brain cope with this bewildering source of new information? Taking his cue from Darwinian selection, Edelman believes that the basic unit in the brain consists of groups or units of neuronal networks consisting of between 50 and 10,000 neurones. There are perhaps a hundred million of such groups. Experience that proves to be of value for the organism is 'mapped' into these neuronal networks. A 'map' is not a representation in the ordinary sense, but an interconnected series of neuronal networks that respond collectively to certain elemental categories or tendencies such as colors in the visual world or a particular situation that triggers a feeling in the emotional world. Edelman calls these categories 'values' because they orient the developing organism toward selecting a limited amount of stimuli from an enormous array of possibilities.
>
> (Cortina 2003)

Throughout development, the brain, in response to the selective stimulation created by experience, repeatedly increases some neural connections and prunes others, so that the surviving neural networks reflect the experiences that have created and repeatedly activated them. Edelman explains:

> A population of variant groups of neurons in a given brain region, comprising neural networks arising by a process of somatic selection, is known as a *primary repertoire*. The genetic code does not provide a specific wiring plan for this repertoire. Rather it imposes a set of constraints on the selection process. Even with such constraints, genetically identical individuals are unlikely to have identical wiring, for selection is epigenetic.
>
> (Edelman 1994[1992]: 83)

He goes on to explain that this primary repertoire is then modified by selective strengthening or weakening of synaptic connections. Edelman continues:

> this mechanism, which underlies memory and a number of other functions, effectively 'carves out' a variety of functioning circuits (with strengthened synapses) from the anatomical network by selection. Such a set of variant functional circuits is called a *secondary repertoire*.
>
> (Edelman 1994[1992]: 85)

However, these surviving neural networks also have to be coordinated among themselves in order for us to develop a coherent and integrated view of the environment and of ourselves. This is achieved by the mechanism called 're-entrant signalling'. Edelman describes this with the example of the visual system of the monkey, which consists of

> over 30 different maps, each with a certain degree of functional segregation (for orientation, colour, movement and so forth) and linked to the others by parallel and reciprocal connections. Re-entrant signalling occurs along these connections. This means that, as groups of neurones are selected in a map, other groups in re-entrantly connected but different maps may also be selected at the same time. Correlation and coordination of such selection events are achieved by re-entrant signalling and by the strengthening of interconnections between the maps within a segment of time.
>
> (Edelman 1994[1992]: 85)

Edelman is clearly arguing that the neurological basis of memory is the particular pattern of neuronal group selection and re-entrant signalling that occurs as a response to repeated interactions with the world: 'Alterations in the synaptic strength of groups in a global mapping provide the biochemical basis of memory' (Edelman 1994[992]: 102).

An integrated conceptual and neurological account of internal working models

Edelman specifically links his ideas with the work of Johnson (1987) on image schemas and others such as Lakoff (1987) who extended this image schematic model into the study of language and semantics.

Edelman suggests that the combination of their work with his provides an integrated biological and conceptual account of human mental functioning. He argues that:

> In the biological view symbols do not get assigned meanings by formal means; instead it is assumed that symbolic structures are meaningful to begin with. This is because categories are determined by bodily structure and by adaptive use as a result of evolution and behaviour. The symbols of cognition must match the conceptual apparatus contained in real brains.
>
> (Edelman 1994[1992]: 239)

He goes on to suggest that image schemas are evolutionarily derived value systems that arise directly out of his own model of neural Darwinism – they match the functioning of the brain.

In addition, Fonagy relates Edelman's model of neural Darwinism with Stern's ideas about early schemata which 'come closest to providing a neuropsychologically valid model of the representation of interpersonal experience' (Fonagy 2001: 119). Schemata are emergent properties of the nervous system and are prototypes which aggregate repeated patterns of lived experience. Stern's 'emergent moments' are the mental consequence of the simultaneous activation of a set of nodes within a network and the resulting strengthening of the connections between these nodes, with each activation automatically constituting a learning process. Neural Darwinism and image schemas may explain the problem Stern posed about cross-modal perception (Stern 1985: 51).

Wilma Bucci (1997) has offered a wide-ranging reconceptualization of psychoanalytic theory in cognitive science terms but does not specifically integrate attachment theory into her model. However, she describes what she terms 'emotion schemas', which seem to be identical to Bowlby's (1988) 'internal working models' in all but name. She proposes that emotion schemas are prototypes that organize new sensory input according to the generalized information stored in the schema and that they are active and dynamic, constantly re-forming in the light of new experiences, just as Bowlby suggested in relation to internal working models. Bucci continues:

The expectations and beliefs built into our emotion schemas determine how we perceive other people, what we expect and how we act. Each person sees all interpersonal experience in the context of the emotion schemas that have been constructed in his life to that point [and continues] whilst the emotion schemas resemble other memory schemas in basic structure and mode of processing, they differ in contents, in particular the dominance of sensory and somatic components and the importance of the interpersonal context in which the schemas are registered and retrieved.

(Bucci 1997: 197)

Having offered a description of emotion schemas that seems to me to differ in no significant way from that of internal working models, Bucci (1997) goes on to make the crucial link to Edelman's theories of neural Darwinism, suggesting that his 'neural maps' provide the neurobiological basis for emotion schemas, and hence, in the terms of attachment theory, for internal working models.

In an echo of the conclusions I drew about the nature of archetypes, I find that understanding the way the mind deals with emotional information requires us to move from a search for structures to an understanding of processes. As Bucci (1997) points out, we need to move from a paradigm in which parts of the brain such as the limbic system are seen as the structures that deal with emotional memories and schemas, to one where the processing of emotion is an activity undertaken by the whole brain and includes cognition, emotion and motivation, which interact together rather than operate independently or even in competition with each other. She continues: 'The multi-component nature of emotions is reflected in their complex cerebral patterning and in the nature of the circuitry linking sensorithalamic, cortical and midbrain structures' (Bucci 1997: 199).

This is a much more dynamic model than the initially influential account of the working of the human brain which was developed by Maclean (1949), who suggested that the processing of emotion takes place in a unified structure, the limbic system, a view that subsequent investigation has called into question. LeDoux (1998) describes in detail the evidence which has been accumulating that contradicts this view, for example, the fact that parts of the limbic system such as the hippocampus are much more involved in cognition than was previously thought. He concludes:

Even as research has shown that classical limbic areas are by no means dedicated to emotion, the theory has persisted. Implicit in such a view is that emotion is a single faculty of mind and that a single unified system of the brain evolved to mediate this faculty. While it is possible that this view is correct, there is little evidence that it is. A new approach to the emotional brain is needed.

(LeDoux 1998: 102)

Conclusions

The integration of neural Darwinism, developmental research and cognitive science does give us, for the first time, a complete account of the internal object. Stern's (1985) account of developmental processes can be seen to be compatible with the image schema as the earliest emergent cognitive structure which underpins conceptual symbolic thought and emotion, and these are rooted in the dynamic, selective biology of Edelman's neural Darwinism.

However, core meanings are based not only on early structures but also on meaning-making processes that constantly sort information from the environment and store it in generalized patterns and rules that govern expectations about the world. While image schemas may function as early emergent Gestalts, organizing frameworks that structure experience but are without any representational content, internal working models function as a store of meaning accumulated by experience, as a body of core meanings which are drawn upon and used but outside conscious awareness. If archetypes can be described in information-processing terms as image schemas, complexes would seem to have many of the information-processing features of internal working models.

In Chapter 5 I want to move on to explore some of the implications which these findings have for psychopathology and clinical practice. In particular, I shall investigate the role of internal working models as defences against painful or unbearable experience. The concepts of internalization and internal working models are frequently misunderstood by those who are first discovering attachment theory, in that they think that there is no room for fantasy and for defensive distortions of reality in the attachment theory model of the psyche. Even Jeremy Holmes (1993) has commented that attachment theory seems to lack some of the richness of the Kleinian world of passionate infantile sexuality. He wrote of

Bowlby: 'An appreciation of the power of phantasy and the complexity of its relationship with external reality is somehow lacking in his work' (Holmes 1993: 6). I disagree with this view, and in Chapter 5 I shall show that internal working models are also the source of defensive fantasies, as well as being formed from real experience. Real experience, when internalized, can be constantly reworked in fantasy, primarily to protect healthy narcissism, the sense of oneself as lovable to others and of value in oneself. Chapter 5 will explore defences in this light.

Trauma and defences

Their roots in relationship

The ideas I have been investigating so far have profound implications for our understanding of unconscious defences. The nature and function of defences are described very differently in psychoanalysis, analytical psychology and attachment theory. I shall explore these respective models and develop an attachment theory perspective in which defences can be seen to evolve out of the earliest patterns of relationship in a child's life. Conscious imagination and unconscious fantasy are constructed as defensive narratives that protect the self from traumatic experiences of abandonment, rejection or cruelty in relationships. Defensive fantasies demonstrate the fact that fantasy does not precede reality but protects the psyche from unbearable reality. First, I will describe the main psychodynamic models of defences in order to clarify what purpose they are thought to serve.

Psychodynamic models of defences

Repression

The earliest Freudian view of repression, the *affect-trauma model*, arose out of Freud's collaboration with Breuer and their attempt to find a psychological explanation for hysterical phenomena. In this model, real trauma plays a key part in the production of symptoms, producing intense emotions and memories which are unacceptable to a person's normal moral standards. Freud described repression as 'a question of things which the patient wished to forget, and therefore intentionally repressed from his conscious thought and inhibited and suppressed' (Freud and Breuer 1893: 10) and it was initially conceived as a form of voluntary dissociation from the consciousness of memories and associated emotions (affects) that were threatening to the individual's standards and ideals (Freud and Breuer 1893).

Repression is thus seen as the pushing away of unacceptable memories, ideas and associated emotions so that these are relegated to the unconscious part of the mind. The emotional excitation remains dammed up outside consciousness. Repression selectively excludes from consciousness those events which might bring to consciousness painful, threatening and distressing emotions which could overwhelm the ego if conscious.

In the *topographical model*, which emerged from 1897 onwards, the emphasis has shifted from the role of actual trauma to the role of instinctual drive. Freud came to the conclusion that his patients' traumatic memories were really wish-fulfilling sexual fantasies. The unconscious was considered to consist of unsatisfied instinctual wishes which derive directly from sexual and aggressive drives. Repression accordingly is a mechanism whereby the subject attempts to repel or confine to the unconscious, representations (thoughts, images, memories) which are bound to an instinct (Freud 1915: 86). Repression occurs when to satisfy an instinct – though likely to be pleasurable in itself – would incur the risk of provoking displeasure because of other requirements.

The topographical model represents a major shift in Freud's thinking towards the view that instinctual drives play a key role in the formation of mental representations so that these store information not only about external events and experiences but also about instinctual wishes. In early infancy, sexual and hostile images, thoughts and feelings towards parents are said to arise universally as an expression of instinctual drives and take the form of the Oedipus complex. Unpleasant emotions of anxiety and, later, guilt trigger the repression mechanisms that keep these mental processes out of consciousness. In the topographical model, experiences or fantasies in later life which have a similar emotional and cognitive content and which therefore would activate unconscious guilt are also repressed; this secondary repression arises from and can be traced back to the original repression of the Oedipus complex. In his 1915 paper on repression, Freud suggested two phases, which he called 'primal repression' and 'repression proper'. Primal repression 'consists in a denial of entry into consciousness to the mental (ideational) presentation of the instinct. This is accompanied by a fixation; the ideational presentation in question persists unaltered from then onwards and the instinct remains attached to it'. Repression proper 'concerns mental derivatives of the repressed instinct-presentation, or such trains of thought as, originating elsewhere, have come into associative connection with it'. There is a clear suggestion in this paper that conscious suppression contributes to repression proper, that there is a voluntary element as well as the involuntary unconscious 'pull' of primal repression (Freud 1915: 148).

The *structural theory* was the third and final formulation of psychic organization which Freud proposed and which he spelt out in full in *The Ego and the Id* (Freud 1923). In the structural theory, Freud concerned himself with describing the organization of mental structures and the relationship between those structures. The *id* is regarded as the reservoir of instinctual, sexual and aggressive drives and wishes and its contents are unconscious. The *ego* is the mental structure that evolves to cope with the demands of external reality and to mediate between the drives, reality and the *superego*. This latter is the mechanism by which mental processes are kept out of consciousness; an unconscious representation is formed of a partly real, partly phantasy, prohibiting and threatening parent, the superego, and this representation is the source of the unconscious guilt which prevents conscious awareness of the 'Oedipal' material. In this model, intrapsychic conflict between the superego, the id and the ego eventually brings about repression, a notion which replaces the former idea of a barrier between conscious and unconscious parts of the mind.

One of the major difficulties with both the topographical and the structural accounts of repression is the assumption that the roots of the Oedipus complex lie in instinctual drives, a problem which also arises with the Kleinian concept of splitting, discussed later. Many present-day Freudians do not accept this account of repression and also consider the unconscious to consist of much more than the dynamically repressed (Fonagy 1999a; Renik 2000).

Psychoanalytic theory has therefore undergone considerable revision, culminating in a *contemporary psychoanalytic model*, in which repression is usually thought of as the intentional keeping out of consciousness of the meaning of a memory rather than the memory of the event itself. Lifting of repression needs to be reconceptualized as a 'change of understanding and feeling in relation to a childhood experience' (Fonagy and Target 1997: 197), rather than the recovery of a previously unavailable memory. This revised view of repression does allow for the possibility that the events themselves could be ordinarily forgotten. It also means that Oedipal conflict is no longer the central issue and cause of repression, although still contributing to it. Oedipal impulses and anxieties can be encompassed within the larger framework of attachment patterns and the development of a healthy narcissism (the development of good and secure self-representations), rather than being seen as expressions of instinctual drive and the main source of the division of the mind into conscious and unconscious parts. Other childhood experiences may have greater significance in contributing to repression, particularly any traumatic event. Anyone who has experienced repeated trauma, whether physical or psychological, may develop a tendency to avoid the emotional significance of experiences, thoughts and fantasies in the past and in the present, and this may be the essence of repression. Such emotional avoidance leaves the person with rigid and outdated schemas of self, object and interpersonal relationships, because they are not constantly updated and revised by new information and experience as a more healthy person's schemas are (Bowlby 1988: 130).

The contemporary psychoanalytic view could be seen as a return to the affect-trauma model of repression combined with features of the structural model; the role of anxiety aroused by traumatic events is recognized rather than the view in the topographical model that instinctual drives play the key role in repression. However, there is a redefinition of what constitutes trauma, with attachment and separation issues playing a central role (Eagle 1995). The contemporary psychoanalytic view of repression also gives a central role to the influence of internal psychic structures, a model which on the surface seems to have some features in common with the superego, id and ego of the structural model. However, in contemporary psychoanalytic models, these internal structures can be considered to be much more closely related to the 'internal working models' of attachment theory rather than to the drive-based psychic structures such as the id.

Splitting, projection and projective identification

Freud did not use the term dissociation but referred instead to 'splitting' of the ego (the agency which has the task of self-preservation by mediating the demands of the id, the superego and

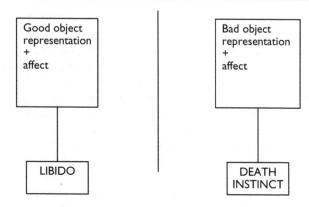

Figure 2 Kleinian concept of splitting

of external reality). He regarded this as a consequence of repression rather than as a different mechanism and described it as the coexistence within a single subject of two contrary and independent attitudes (Freud 1940[1938]: 204). *A Dictionary of Kleinian Thought* (Hinshelwood 1989) has no reference to the term 'dissociation', but only to the term 'splitting'; it was predominantly Melanie Klein who developed this concept of splitting as a fundamental part of her model of psychic mechanisms. Klein extended Freud's concept of splitting to include splitting of the object as well as of the ego, so that in her model, the mind would contain ego + object representations with a particular affect tone, kept separate from other clusters of ego + object representations with a different affect tone (Klein 1946: 6).

According to Klein, splitting is a different process from repression and is conceived as an earlier developmental mechanism, which therefore may exert an influence on the form that later repression takes. Splitting is described by Kleinians as a more severe defence, dividing the mind into two parts with object relationship and ego in each part, and each separate relationship coexisting side by side (Figure 2).

A fundamental principle of this model is that splitting is not primarily a mechanism for keeping memories of real events out of consciousness, but rather, for keeping anxiety derived from the death instinct out of consciousness. The death instinct is conceived of as a separate instinct from libido and one which is essentially destructive, with the aim 'to undo connections and so to destroy things. In the case of the destructive instinct we may suppose that its final aim is to lead what is living into an inorganic state. For this reason we call it the death instinct' (Freud 1940[1938]: 161).

The problem is that Klein developed this model from her clinical work with patients with severe clinical symptomatology; she observed phenomena such as resistance (in which the analyst's interpretations are strongly rejected), acting out (in which the patient resorts to non-verbal means of communication such as missing sessions, prolonged silences or destructive behaviour outside the analytic room) and various other negative therapeutic reactions, and then derived a developmental model from these clinical patterns, a model which was assumed to apply to normal as well as abnormal psychological development. Dissociative mechanisms which she observed in her adult and child patients were assumed to originate in the first few months of life, a phase which she described as the 'paranoid schizoid' position, in which she suggested that the infant experiences external reality in a polarized and split way, as either totally gratifying and good or totally persecutory and bad. *A Dictionary of Kleinian Thought* (Hinshelwood 1989: 419) states: 'The splitting of parts of the self becomes, in the course of development, a split between the conscious and the unconscious – i.e. repression'.

In the Kleinian model, split-off unconscious phantasies prevent accurate perception of external reality. External events are perceived and reorganized within the framework of the relevant pre-existing unconscious phantasy and frequently distorted by it (Perlow 1995: 157). Such distortion would affect memories as well as perception, and Kleinian analysts focus much less on patients' memories as representations of real events and more on them as expressions of unconscious phantasies and therefore of the presumed instinctual drive which the phantasy is supposed to express. In Chapter 4, I have reviewed the evidence that innate and complex mental imagery does not arise in the first six months of life as Kleinian theory suggests.

However, if the notion of instinct-based unconscious phantasy is discarded, there remains the aspect of Kleinian theory which does correspond to cognitive science accounts of the mind, and that is the view that pre-existing schemas organize perception. Empirical research suggests that cognitive schemas are internalized and generalized representations of past experience (Blaxton 1989; Hamann 1990; Schacter 1996). Fonagy (1999a) has reviewed the evidence which suggests that schemas of self–other relationships are also stored implicitly, as a network of unconscious expectations or mental models that organize interpersonal behaviour but are not consciously accessible. These mental models are derived from accumulated past experience but stored independently and separately from discrete autobiographical memories (Fonagy 1999a). Many therapists do find their patients have mental representations grouped into clusters around a common emotional tone and 'split' from each other, but there are developmental accounts of this, such as that of the internal working model, which in no way depend upon the Kleinian explanation that these splits arise from instinctual drives.

Projection and projective identification are concepts closely linked to that of splitting. Hinshelwood (1989) summarized the range of ways in which good or bad versions of internal objects and parts of the self are projected into others and related to outside oneself, pointing out the difficulty in a precise distinction between these terms (Hinshelwood 1989: 387).

Dissociation

Dissociation is the term that Jung usually used (although sometimes the term 'splitting' is used instead). One major difference between the Jungian use of this concept and the Kleinian meaning of the term 'splitting' is that Jungian dissociation is not rooted in drive theory; it is a description of structural divisions in the psyche, but a quite different structural division from that of Freud's structural model. However, there is an added complication in that Fordham, who modified Jungian theory and applied it to infant development, tended to use Kleinian models and terminology, such as splitting, integrating these into Jungian theory without always fully untangling the theoretical incompatibilities of the two terms (Knox 1997).

In Chapter 4 I explored Jung's use of the term dissociation in relation to Janet's (1925[1919]) formulation of the concept, showing that it gives rise to complexes, splinter psyches which are dissociated from each other. The extent to which Jung's account of dissociation has its origins in Janet's ideas has been carefully investigated by John Haule (1999). This is a very different use of Janet's ideas from that of the information-processing model of contemporary clinical psychology, where dissociation is considered to be an altered state of consciousness which gives rise to post-traumatic stress disorder (PTSD) and, in its most extreme form, to dissociative identity disorder. For example, van der Kolk and Fisler (1995) showed that trauma leads to abnormal encoding of sensory and affective elements of the traumatic experience and that, in PTSD, these are retrieved as visual, olfactory, affective, auditory and kinaesthetic experiences, which are dissociated from any coherent semantic component. Brewin *et al.* (1996) have also proposed that, in traumatic conditions, intense emotion alters the way in which mental representations are formed, so that situationally accessible memories or representations are formed, encoded and stored separately from verbally accessible memories. Verbally accessible memories are representations of a person's conscious experience of a trauma and these can 'in principle be deliberately retrieved from the store of autobiographical experiences' (Brewin *et al.* 1996: 676). Situationally accessible memories (SAMs) cannot be accessed deliberately, but resurface automatically when the person is in a context in which the physical features or meaning are similar to those of the traumatic situation. SAMs tend to be highly detailed, repetitive memories (flashbacks) that are accompanied by the emotional and physiological changes experienced during the trauma. They suggest that these two types of mental representations account for many of the clinical phenomena associated with post-traumatic stress disorder (Brewin *et al.* 1996).

However, the Jungian model of dissociation is closer to this model than at first appears, in that its roots lie in Janet's recognition that when people experience intense emotions, memories cannot be transformed into a narrative. Janet wrote that under these circumstances a person is 'unable to make a recital which we call narrative memory, and yet he remains confronted by the difficult situation' (Janet 1925[1919]: 660). He suggested that this leads to a failure to integrate the traumatic memories which remain split off from ordinary consciousness, a view which is supported by the research of van der Kolk and Fisler (1995).

Whereas repression is a division between conscious and unconscious functioning of the mind, in dissociation, one set of conscious and unconscious representations is kept separate from another. Emotion is included in the functioning of these dissociated parts of the mind called 'complexes', which are 'feeling-toned groups of representations' in the unconscious. Jacobi (1959) emphasizes that 'the complexes are impressive indicators not only of the "divisibility" or "dissociability" of the psyche but also of the relative independence of the fragments, which may amount to complete psychic disintegration in all its variants' (Jacobi 1959: 12). For Jung psychological difficulties do not arise from the influence of repressed childhood memories, but from a difficulty in the present which activates a dissociated part of the mind, a complex, which then dominates mental functioning inappropriately and without self-reflection.

This brief survey shows that it is only in early Freudian theory, in the affect-trauma model, that the influence of emotion on memory is considered to be the key mechanism. In contrast, in contemporary psychoanalytic theory it is the influence of emotion on the formation and accessibility of self, object and interpersonal schemas (or working models) which is considered to be crucial.

In Kleinian theory it is 'innate' processes called instinctual drives which distort memory and perception by means of the phantasies which give expression to the drives. These are postulated to be active in adults as well as children, so it is not memories of childhood fantasies which distort memory and perception in adulthood, but the continuing activity of the instinctual drives and the unconscious fantasies they give rise to. The purpose of defences such as splitting and projection is to protect 'good' from 'bad' self and object representations.

In Jungian theory it is dissociated schemas, called complexes, each with an archetypal nucleus which influence and interact with perception and memory; the complex consists of innate expectation, mental representations and emotions. Present experience is interpreted and responded to in the light of the complex which is controlling attention.

An attachment theory model of defences: trauma, defences and affect regulation

An attachment theory model of defences has some features in common with each of these differing frameworks, although some authors have argued that it is closest to the contemporary psychoanalytic perspective. These similarities will be explored in more detail later. However, in attachment theory, the purpose of defences is very different from the role that they are thought to serve within the frameworks I have just summarized. In attachment theory, the main purpose of defences is *affect regulation*, a view introduced in a classic article by Sroufe and Waters and widely accepted by contemporary attachment theorists (Sroufe and Waters 1977; Goldberg 2000: 136–9). The main mechanism for achieving this in infancy is *distance regulation*, a range of behavioural strategies which is most evident in young infants, for example in the Strange Situation. In adults 'secondary strategies at the representational level can be seen to parallel these infant behavioural strategies' so that intrapsychic mechanisms can be thought of as a symbolic form of distance regulation, a way of keeping distressing memories and ideas at a safe distance from consciousness (Dozier *et al.* 2001: 63). Bowlby described this intrapsychic form of distance regulation as *defensive exclusion* (Bowlby 1980: 45).

In both cases it is the relationship to key attachment figures which is the central focus for feelings of security and a sense of comfort and well-being or the alternative experience of insecurity and the distress this causes, so that affect regulation is inextricably linked to the actual experience of relationship and to the internal working models built up from that experience. This is one of the most crucial contributions of attachment theory to a contemporary psychodynamic understanding of the intrapsychic world, which can no longer be considered a solipsistic closed system, insulated from the effects of actual experience and the impact of other people's intrapsychic states: it is a relational and interpersonal unconscious (Schore 1994; Brown and Harris 1978). Holmes (2001) places the roots of this interpersonal unconscious in the evolutionary pressures, writing that 'where infants are exposed to predators and the only guarantee of security is the bond to a parent, there would be strong selective pressure towards attachment behaviours' (Holmes 2001: 24).

Defences as higher order internal working models and their role in appraisal

At first sight it might be easy to reify defences as described in attachment theory and so to fail to appreciate the intrapsychic process that underpin defensive patterns of behaviour, relationship, thought and emotion. In Chapter 4, I highlighted Cortina's view of the central role that appraisal plays in the processing of information in general and defensive processes in particular. He writes: 'Appraising, selecting and interpreting experience is not a function of an agency of the mind such as the id or the ego or superego; *it is what the brain does'* (Cortina 2003, original emphasis). Internal working models play a key role in this process of appraisal, especially in relation to appraisal of the degree of safety or danger in the world around us, a process as essential to psychological as it is to physical survival.

It is vital to recognize that distance regulation and defensive exclusion are the behavioural and emotional manifestations of the operation of internal working models, which contain information that the parent (or other key attachment figure) avoids intimacy or is alternately overwhelming and rejecting. These internal working models also contain self-representations and representations of the pattern of relationship between infant and parent, including the defensive patterns that have emerged as a means of avoiding intense distress – in other words as a means of affect regulation. The reader should bear in mind that, when I describe a behavioural strategy, there is always an intrapsychic model that motivates the behaviour, which should therefore never be thought of as a mindless automatic behavioural response to a stimulus.

The Strange Situation demonstrates clearly the behavioural strategies that infants acquire in order to cope with the distress that is caused by a parent who is unavailable or unpredictable and unreliable. Dozier *et al.* (2001) describe this:

> Rather than directly seeking out and obtaining comfort from the caregiver, such infants employ secondary strategies that involve the deactivation or hyperactivation of the attachment system. The deactivation of the attachment system is characterized by avoidance of the caregiver when the infant is distressed or needy. Hyperactivation of the attachment system is characterized by preoccupation with the caregiver (at times when most other infants would not seek out the caregiver) and resistance to the caregiver's ministrations.
>
> (Dozier *et al.* 2001: 63)

Distance regulation is an effective strategy for the regulation of affect because emotion is so dependent on the relationship with the caregiver. The intrapsychic and the interpersonal are inextricable in early infancy. Holmes (1993) points out that both the avoidant and the preoccupied (or ambivalent) strategies can be formulated in terms of dilemmas 'arising out of the need to get close and the imagined dangers of doing so: rejection, abandonment or intrusion'

(Holmes 1993: 150). Avoidant infants have learnt that the attachment figure may reject their advances and so suppress their needs and distance themselves from the caregiver. Avoidant infants communicate directly with mother only when they are feeling well. When distressed, they do not seek contact but mask negative emotion and engage in self-soothing behaviour (Cassidy 2001). The ambivalent child fears that the attachment figure may either fail to respond or will intrude in a way that she cannot control; she therefore clings and insists on controlling the caregiver's response. It is as though the infant has to take on more than its share of the burden of maintaining the connection (Bretherton 1985) and lacks confidence that the caregiver will be available if needed. Disorganized attachment is a third pattern of insecure attachment that has been identified and is usually considered to be the most severe. There is no organized behavioural strategy because these infants have experienced caregivers who are themselves the source of threat to the infant who is therefore faced with the terrible dilemma of seeking comfort from the person who is frightening him or her. Neither proximity seeking nor proximity avoiding is a solution (Cassidy 2001).

Holmes (1993) offers some innovative reflections on the nature of unconscious processes and their relationship to these patterns of behaviour, suggesting that behavioural strategies such as distance regulation serve to maintain attachments in the face of relational forces that threaten to disrupt them and describing this as the 'behavioral unconscious'. The body (and hence, I would add, the degree of physical distance from other 'safe' bodies) is 'the intermediate zone between the mind and the Other' (Holmes 2001: 25). Goldberg offers a more detailed account of the behavioural strategies involved, describing avoidant patterns as a form of deactivation which attempts to suppress information associated with attachment needs, including affect, while ambivalent patterns reflect hyperactivation, in which there is an exaggeration of attachment behaviours and emotions (Goldberg 2000: 137).

Links between attachment based and psychodynamic models of intrapsychic defences

Attachment theory suggests that, throughout childhood development and into adult life, experiences of relationships are internalized and stored as generalized patterns in implicit memory, in the form of internal working models (see Chapter 4). These guide expectations of subsequent relationships, while a range of studies have demonstrated the consistency of the patterns of attachment established in early infancy as shown in the Strange Situation (Cassidy 2001; Karen 1998). The behavioural regulation of affect evident in early infancy becomes internalized as a part of this process of formation of internal working models. Fonagy (2001) points out that this is not a new idea, writing:

> The notion that psychic functions may be internalized from primary object relationships is present in the writings of a number of psychoanalytic authors . . . For example, Bion's (1959, 1962a) model of containment also assumes that the infant internalizes the function of transformation exercised by the caregiver, and through this acquires the capacity to contain or regulate his own negative affective states.
>
> (Fonagy 2001: 164–5)

Once again, affect regulation is placed at the heart of intrapsychic processes. I suggested earlier that intrapsychic defences mirror the behavioural defences of early infancy and the most obvious manifestation of this is the defensive exclusion that Bowlby himself described. This calls into question Holmes's suggestion that the unconscious of attachment theory is a behavioural unconscious (Holmes 2001: 24). The patterns of relationship of early infancy, including defensive patterns of distance regulation, are internalized and stored as internal working models, which are schematic patterns, stored in implicit memory, a format that renders them inaccessible to consciousness. However, they are not merely procedural 'habits' but they are fully symbolic, representational and intrapsychic models which exert a powerful organizing influence not only on behaviour but also on conscious beliefs, attitudes, emotions and desires, while remaining unconscious in themselves. The core internal working models of relationships can be elicited by means of the second major attachment research tool, the Adult Attachment Interview developed by Mary Main (Main and Goldwyn 1995). From an evolutionary perspective, Susan Goldberg suggests that 'the ability to construct such representations evolved because they confer a survival advantage. They allow individuals to selectively attend to information, predict future events and construct plans' (Goldberg 2000: 150). Internal working models play a crucial role in the constant evaluation of the world which is essential for survival; this process of appraisal also requires an imaginative exploration of possible future events not only consciously but also unconsciously, so that internal working models play a major part in unconscious fantasy.

Internal working models therefore do not bear any clear relationship to Freud's central idea that unconscious contents are always the result of an active process of repression. However, the concept of the internal working model does have much in common with Jung's model of the complex, as I described in Chapter 4. Like complexes, internal working models are based on the mechanism of dissociation (or splitting) rather than repression, in that a 'vertical' split keeps some conscious and unconscious contents separate from others, while repression reflects the operation of a 'horizontal' split in which conscious attention is kept away from certain disturbing or distressing unconscious contents.

However, the concept of defensive exclusion may have more in common with repression than at first appears, in that it may offer the basis for a hierarchy of defensive strategies and mechanisms, ranging from conscious suppression, through unconscious repression to splitting and dissociation. Defensive avoidance of painful experiences, thoughts and memories may initially be conscious and voluntary (suppression), but gradually become unconscious and automatic (repression), so that eventually whole clusters of associated mental representations become unconscious islands, disconnected from each other and from conscious awareness (dissociation). The view that repression originates in conscious suppression is strongly advocated by Erdelyi (1995), who draws on one of Freud's earliest definitions of repression to support this: 'it was a question of things which the patient wished to forget, and therefore intentionally repressed from his conscious thought and inhibited and suppressed (Freud and Breuer [1893]1955)'. Erdelyi suggests that 'a conscious defensive operation, through repeated use, may gradually become automatic and essentially unconscious in deployment' (Erdelyi 1995: 15). The suggestion that persistent repression may lead eventually to the more complete separation of mental contents from each other that occurs in dissociation is lent support by Bretherton (1995):

> Although defensive exclusion protects the individual from experiencing unbearable mental pain, confusion, or conflict, it

is bound to interfere with the accommodation of internal working models to external reality. Indeed a number of clinical studies reviewed in *Separation* (e.g., Cain and Fast, 1972) suggest that defensive exclusion leads to a split in internal working models.

(Bretherton 1995: 68)

Other attachment researchers also highlight the fact that defensive exclusion eventually leads to 'the development of segregated or dissociated memory systems for the loss experience. Because these memories still exist, albeit in an unintegrated form, they can continue to influence emotion and behaviour without the person's understanding how or why' (Fraley and Shaver 1999: 742). The similarity between this account of segregated internal working models and Jung's description of complexes is striking. Jung wrote that a complex is 'subject to the control of the conscious mind to only a limited extent, and therefore behaves like an animated foreign body in the sphere of consciousness' (Jung 1960[1934]: 96).

Are these defensive strategies successful in regulating affect so that the infant does not experience too much distress? Fonagy *et al.* (1995) point out that all forms of insecure attachment are defensive compromises 'in which either intimacy (avoidant/dismissing) or autonomy (resistant/preoccupied) appears to be sacrificed for the sake of retaining physical proximity to the caregiver incapable of containing the infant's affect' (Fonagy *et al.* 1995: 243). While the avoidant pattern may permit an infant to disengage from a painful situation, the resistant pattern may attract the attention of an emotionally preoccupied parent, for example, making a depressed or withdrawn mother 'come to life'. The avoidant pattern seems to carry a price for the conscious avoidance of attention to painful ideas and experiences. Eagle (1995) suggests that 'the low anxiety and low distress reported by the individual employing a repressive style are belied by the relatively high levels of physiological arousal shown, particularly during stress' and suggests that this may also be the case with avoidant patterns of attachment (Eagle 1995: 144). He also suggests that the preoccupied pattern of attachment is more maladaptive and less successful than the avoidant pattern, in that these people cannot shut out distressing thoughts and feelings and instead try not to show others how distressed they actually are.

Bowlby himself mainly explored defensive exclusion but he did not emphasize the fact that the defensive behaviour always has its roots in internal working models in which the accumulated experience of defensive patterns of relationship between child and parent is stored. He also did not investigate other defensive strategies such as the construction of narratives in imagination and fantasy which can diminish anxiety and regulate emotion, in that they provide alternative and more acceptable symbolic significance to experience. This aspect of fantasy will be discussed more fully in the next section.

Trauma and the defensive function of fantasy

Instinctual drive theory, which proposes that unconscious fantasy is a direct expression of instinctual drives, is a theory which many psychoanalysts believe in with great passion, partly because it provides an explanation for the distortions of external reality which are so evident in our clinical work. We do need to be able to account for the way in which internal objects are formed and why they can differ so much from the actual people, usually parents, who have played such a central part in the formation of our internal world. The psychoanalytic model of instinctual drives, originally propounded by Freud and emphasized by Klein, gives us an easy answer by proposing that the external reality is relatively unimportant and that the magical or terrifying 'good' or 'bad' internal object arises as a direct expression of the 'life' and 'death' instincts. Thus Melanie Klein said that 'the child anticipates, by reason of his own cannibalistic and sadistic impulses, such punishment as castration, being cut into pieces, eaten up, etc. and lives in perpetual dread of them' (Klein 1927: 155); one of her closest supporters, Joan Riviere, said that 'psychoanalysis is Freud's discovery of what goes on in the imagination . . . it has no concern with anything else, it is not concerned with the real world' (quoted in Holmes 1993: 130).

However, attachment theory can offer us a very different way of conceptualizing fantasy, based upon the key features of the internal working model and the defensive processes, which I have described. Unfortunately, Bowlby himself did not really investigate the concept of fantasy because he saw it as inextricably a part of the Kleinian model with its focus on instinctual drive as the source of fantasy. He took great pains to convey his firm and passionate conviction that real-life experience plays a key role in the creation of psychological distress and psychopathology and remained critical throughout his life of psychoanalysts who attributed these phenomena to the distortions produced by unconscious fantasy. In addition, Bowlby's model of defensive processes centred on defensive exclusion, and this view of defences as essentially avoidant did not provide much scope for an exploration of the constructive aspects of fantasy, the imaginative narratives and models that a child unconsciously builds in order to make sense of experiences and to reduce the distress that some memories may cause. However, in *Separation: Anxiety and Anger*, Bowlby (1973) did investigate the extent to which a child's imperfect understanding of the world and its dangers might lead to 'imaginary' fears. He reminds us that alertness to environmental cues that indicate danger is a vital survival strategy, suggesting that 'if living beings are to survive, there can be no great margin for error' (Bowlby 1973: 156), so that so-called imaginary fears can be seen as defensive narratives constructed to define specific dangers and to avoid them:

> Thus, when the bathwater goes down the plughole, how is a toddler to know he will not go down too? When, later, he hears tales of robbers and red Indians intercepting coaches or robbing mail-trains, how is he to know that he and his family may not be the next victims? The very great difficulty a child has in appraising at all accurately the degree of danger in which at any moment he may stand accounts, it is argued, for a much larger proportion of the so-called imaginary fears of childhood than is often supposed.
>
> (Bowlby 1973: 157)

The purpose of these imaginative explanations that children (and adults) construct is to provide a meaningful narrative that can then be used to predict and avoid danger. Bowlby gives an example of a small boy who ran hurriedly away each time a photographer tried to take his picture; later it was revealed that he thought he was about to be killed each time he heard the word 'shoot'.

This construction of narratives serves a protective and defensive purpose by ordering experience into patterns so that the world does not seem to be a place where dangers occur which the child can neither predict nor control. This is an unconscious as well as a conscious process, in that the vulnerability, which is part of being a small child dependent on adults, often leads to experiences of helplessness and humiliation. This highlights a crucial issue, namely the fact that fantasy is a normal activity and a healthy part of psychic development, indeed serving an essential role in the construction of the child's growing sense of identity and relationship. Infantile illusions of magical omnipotence play a key role in the creation of a healthy narcissism, as Winnicott (1975[1951]) pointed out. Eliot (1935) said that humankind cannot bear very much reality and Winnicott's work adds a developmental perspective to this, showing that we all need to be protected from the pain of awareness of our separateness until we have achieved the psychic capacity to tolerate that knowledge (Winnicott 1975[1951]). Fantasy can contribute a necessary defence against intrusions of reality that we are not yet equipped to deal with. Fonagy (2001: 111) points out that attachment theory does not seem to have a place for the concept of infantile grandiosity or omnipotence, but I would suggest that these can be understood, not as primary motivational systems but rather as defensive fantasies against the humiliating sense of helplessness that an infant experiences when a parent is insensitive or abusive. It is humiliating because the infant feels that his or her normal emotional needs are unwanted by the parent and therefore something to be ashamed of, an experience which leaves a deep narcissistic wound. Kohut (1972) suggests that this injured narcissism calls forth both rage and fantasies of grandiosity to protect the ego from the shameful awareness of rejected dependence.

This approach can also offer an attachment theory perspective on the Oedipus complex, a concept which Bowlby largely neglected, perhaps because it seemed so inextricably bound up with instinctual drive theory. However, it is possible to offer a new understanding of the Oedipus complex in terms of Oedipal patterns of attachment. This reflects an idea, which seems to be gaining ground, that the manifestations of attachment may change with growth and development. In one of a series of articles reviewing the concept of internal working models, Bretherton (1999) takes Bowlby's (1969) notion of 'a goal-directed partnership' to suggest that the nature of attachment itself may change with development and that a more sophisticated kind of attachment may become possible when the child's attachment plans become infused with 'some insight into his mother's goals and motives' (Bretherton 1999; Bowlby 1969: 267–8). In the same series of articles, Nelson (1999) argues that 'one could expect changes not only in the quality of the attachment relationship itself, but also in the understanding of that relationship under different conditions of discursive interactions during the childhood years' (Nelson 1999: 249).

How does this help us to develop an attachment theory framework for understanding the core anxieties and defences of the Oedipal stage of development? A key part of such development for a small child is the growing awareness that his or her parents have a sexual relationship with each other which excludes the child, and this awareness would form a very important part of the insight into the mother's goals and intentions to which Bowlby (1969) refers, and into the change in quality of the attachment relationship which Nelson (1999) proposes. This awareness and the accompanying desires and fears of the Oedipal stage could therefore be considered as a developmentally driven modification of the attachment relationship. New internal working models would be formed, containing new representations of the key attachment figures, their relationships with each other, and new representations of self in relation to each parent and these new internal working models would underpin Oedipal patterns of attachment and defences.

Furthermore, Fonagy (1999b) specifically links Kohut's (1972) view that narcissism has its own developmental pathway with an attachment perspective on the Oedipus complex, suggesting that Kohut

> characterized the Oedipus complex as the child's reaction to the parent's failure to enjoy and participate empathically in the child's growth. Unempathic parents are likely to react to their oedipal child with counterhostility or counterseduction. Such reactions may stimulate destructive aggression and isolated sexual fixation. Kohut identified castration anxiety and penis envy, as Bowlby might have been inclined to do as imposed from outside rather than being the consequence of a constitutional predisposition to Oedipal experiences.
>
> (Fonagy 1999b: 611)

The key role of the parental attitude to the child's Oedipal feelings highlights another key feature of an attachment theory model of the defensive role of fantasy, namely that of intergenerational transmission of attachment patterns. The research done by Steele *et al.* (1986) has demonstrated clearly that the internal working models of the parents powerfully influence the growing child's internal working models, reflected in the patterns of attachment which the child shows; a mother who has a dismissive rating on the Adult Attachment Interview, a pattern which demonstrates an avoidance of emotionally painful memories about her own life, is most likely to have a child who shows an avoidant pattern of attachment (Steele *et al.* 1996).

As part of the defensive function of fantasy, memories may also be re-examined and reconstructed. This really draws us towards the conclusion that memory can become fantasy and fantasy can become memory. In a symposium on the subject of recovered memory, Fonagy (1997) made a similar point:

> We are setting up truth against falsehood, history against phantasy, fact against desire . . . [but] these pairs of opposites do not exist independently . . . the dialectic of fact and desire is that fact makes desire and then desire makes fact, in an interminable sequence of events and thoughts that are repeated throughout life.
>
> (Fonagy 1997: 126)

As part of this process, wishes, desires and fears not only influence and distort the way we experience events but also form part of that experience, and so themselves become incorporated into the memories of those events. Internal working models, the unconscious patterns of beliefs and expectations about relationships that are built up through the process of internalization are not only a form of memory, but also a new way of conceptualizing unconscious fantasy. The child's own emotions and the imaginative narratives that he or she constructs to make sense of the world or to maintain a positive sense of identity become included in unconscious 'working models' as they develop. Eagle (1995) also draws important implications for the concept of fantasy from the idea of multiple and often conflicting internal working models. He suggests that 'some working models may represent idealized representations that reflect the operations of defence and the fantasy of what the child would have liked the relationship with the caregiver to be, rather than the actual caregiving experience' (Eagle 1995: 127). Accurate memories of past experience may coexist alongside both defensive and wish-fulfilling internal working models which offer a conflicting intrapsychic picture. Fantasy can take the form of unconscious narratives which offer imaginative solutions to the dilemmas and problems that life creates, a form of unconscious playful rehearsal of a range of possible attitudes and actions. Unconscious fantasies therefore serve a normal developmental function, opening up new avenues for the child's developing psyche to explore.

However, this exploratory function of fantasy, which is one of the mechanisms by which an infant constantly unconsciously appraises the degree of safety or danger in the world around him or her, may also play a central role when a child is abused, particularly if the abuser is the person to whom the child is most attached, such as one or other of the parents. To feel hated by a parent is intolerable and the fear, humiliation and sense of helplessness are likely to produce profound narcissistic damage, unless this can be modified by a degree of omnipotent fantasy. For example, a child who is subject to random and unpredictable violence from a parent will feel not only pain and terror but also a sense of complete helplessness, with no power to influence the parent's behaviour or to have any control over the situation. In addition, without any apparent cause for the parent's cruelty, the child has to face the intolerable fact that the parent is at that moment hostile, malevolent and sadistic towards the child. I think that for any child to feel this is unbearable and that it may be preferable in that situation for children to construct a belief or fantasy that they have done something to cause their parent to behave in this sadistic way; such an imaginative belief would allow children to retain some sense of cause and effect, some belief that they actually do have some control over the situation because they did something wrong which provoked this violent response. The belief that they caused the parent's violence by some bad behaviour also allows children to retain the belief that their parent will love them again, that it is the bad behaviour that is being punished and not that the parent really hates the child.

This kind of defensive belief becomes part of the unconscious 'working model' of relationships with key attachment figures and may emerge in relationships in adult life in the form of an unconscious fantasy that the person is responsible for others' bad behaviour and should be punished for it; it might be quite easy for this person to become a battered spouse as a kind of enactment of the unconscious fantasy and/or memory. The internal working model produces a pattern of implicit beliefs and expectations that determine, for example, the choice of a partner and the nature of the relationship that subsequently develops. A person's unconscious fantasy that he or she is to blame if her partner is abusive could evoke the same belief in the partner and easily lead to the re-creation of the childhood experience, since 'one may unconsciously seek out objects who resonate with early attachment figures and patterns of relating, that, however unsatisfactory they may have been, provided the only felt security one experienced' (Eagle 1995: 142).

Projection and projective identification

The example just given shows that projection and projective identification can be understood, not as purely intrapsychic mechanisms but as interactional processes. They are the consequence of the activation of internal working models which not only organize and often distort perception of external reality but also exert a strong influence on a person's own behaviour and the cues they emit to others. Eagle (1995) suggests that in analysis patients' unconscious expectations produce patterns of behaviour, often quite subtle, that usually evoke certain predictable responses from others and that analysts need to recognize that their own countertransference has been evoked in this way in order to interpret the unconscious expectations that lie behind patients' behaviour and its effect on the analysts themselves. Fonagy (2001: 87) also highlights the interactional nature of projective identification, writing that projective identification is not a truly internal process; it involves the 'object', who may experience it as manipulation, seduction or a myriad of other forms of psychic influence. Spillius (1994) has suggested the use of the term 'evocatory projective identification' to designate instances in which the recipient of projective identification is put under pressure to have the feelings appropriate to the projector's fantasy.

The implication of this approach to projection and projective identification is that they are defensive internal working models, rooted in the person's past experience and are not manifestations of the death instinct, which was one way in which Klein understood projective identification. However, Klein (1933), and more particularly Bion (1959), did fully recognize the interpersonal and communicative aspects of projective identification and the aim to 'introduce into the object a state of mind, as a means of communicating with it about this mental state' (Hinshelwood 1989: 184)

Once again, attachment theory has demonstrated its remarkable capacity to act as a bridge between hermeneutic and empirical understanding of the human psyche, in evolving research tools that can demonstrate the impact of a parent's unconscious meaning on that of his or her child. Studies have shown that it is the parent's internal world, not purely his or her behaviour, that is the formative influence on the child's unconscious experience of relationship, demonstrated in the child's pattern of attachment. Fonagy *et al.* (1991) have shown that the parent's working model of attachment, as measured on the Adult Attachment Interview before the infant's birth, correlates with the infant's subsequent security of attachment to that parent, demonstrated in the Strange Situation. Furthermore, each parent transmits his or her internal working model independently of the other, so that the child develops and maintains distinguishable sets of expectations in relation to each parent (Fonagy *et al.* 1991). Unconscious communication certainly is a reality and I think it is very confusing for patients if their perceptions of these unconscious pressures are misinterpreted as entirely a product of their own unconscious phantasies. The individuation process needs us to recognize that we all internalize the unconscious of others, which can be experienced as an alien, but at the same time an internal, psyche.

Jung anticipated this development in psychoanalysis and attachment theory when he recognized the real effect that one person's unconscious can have on another and hence the intersubjective nature of analytic work. He was the first to propose that analysts should first be analysed themselves in order to minimize the impact of their own unconscious conflicts on the analysand, although he recognized that this could be only partially achieved. The implication of this for analytic work will be discussed more fully in Chapter 7, but the point here is to highlight Jung's awareness of the reality of the impact of one person's unconscious processes on another, such as the influence of the parental unconscious on the child, writing that 'I have frequently observed children who were particularly influenced by certain unconscious tendencies in the parents' (Jung 1920: para. 1793).

As we have already seen, Fraiberg *et al.* (1975) so evocatively wrote: 'In every nursery there are ghosts. These are the visitors from the unremembered pasts of the parents; the uninvited guests at the christening'. A less poetic term to describe the mechanism by which the parental ghosts are incorporated into the infant's unconscious is transgenerational transmission. This transmission of unconscious parental processes may on occasion give rise to massive defences against what is experienced as an alien intrusion, if the parental unconscious is very threatening. Alicia Lieberman has also explored the processes by which babies 'become the carriers of the parents' unconscious fears, impulses, and other repressed or disowned parts of themselves' and how these 'negative attributions become an integral part of the child's sense of self' (Lieberman 1999). This process may begin even *in utero*, as Rosenfeld (1987) suggests, describing the powerful influence or 'osmotic overflow' of a mother's experiences and memories, which are unbearable to her and so denied, to her unborn foetus (Rosenfeld 1987: 185). Some tentative empirical support for this comes from Piontelli's (1992) ultrasound studies of foetuses whom she then observed through early childhood, noting that physical trauma during pregnancy seemed to be reflected in the later child-hood patterns of behaviour. Piontelli also suggested that maternal anxiety could have been a factor in the behaviour of some of the foetuses she observed (Piontelli 1992: 240).

There are some clinical accounts of extreme defences against invasion by the alien other. Affeld-Niemayer (1995) describes victims of incestuous sexual abuse whose loss of instinctual experience and reality sense reflects an extreme regression to a primary undifferentiated stage of development in which 'the identity of the victim is taken over by that of the aggressor and become petrified in a form of mimicry'. I think this kind of paralysis may reflect the fact that paedophiles often seize on any kind of excitement in the child, regardless of its nature, as an invitation or permission for sexual abuse. Wheeley (1992) described her work with a patient whose mother unconsciously communicated murderous feelings towards her, which the patient then communicated by projective identification to the analyst so that she at times felt murderous to her patient. Fonagy (2001) suggests that projective identification is the main defence against the intolerable experience of hostile caregiving, which forces the child to internalize aspects of the caregiver that the child cannot then integrate. The alien unassimi-lated parts can be dealt with only by forcing them into others (Fonagy 2001: 88).

Grandiosity and archetypal defences

The suggestion that infantile fantasies of grandiosity and omni-potence emerge as defences against too painful an awareness of the reality that, as a small child, one is helpless, vulnerable and dependent has considerable implications for a Jungian view of psychic defences. Fonagy (2001) suggests that Kohut's (1972) view of grandiosity as a defence against a narcissistic injury can be described in attachment theory terms as forming one part of a dual and polarized internal working model:

> One component contains a set of omnipotent expectations, based on the child's view of the parent's capacities mixed with infantile omnipotence, and the other component is one of total helplessness and enfeeblement, the expectations of an infant facing an unempathic caregiver.
>
> (Fonagy 2001: 109)

This description of a polarized internal working model, containing omnipotent fantasies that defend against actual or feared rejection and humiliation, has considerable similarities, but also some differences from the concept proposed by Kalsched (1996) of archetypal defences which are activated by unbearable trauma. Kalsched highlights the vital protective role that dissociative defences play when a person is threatened with intolerable trauma, psychic pain or anxiety which are severe enough to bring about psychic disintegration, or 'the destruction of the personal spirit'. He suggests that trauma produces a fragmentation of consciousness in which one part of the personality regresses to an infantile state and another part progresses in a false and omnipotent adaptation to the outside world. The regressed part of the personality is usually represented as a vulnerable innocent child or animal, while the progressed part appears in dreams as a powerful benevolent or malevolent great being who protects or persecutes its vulnerable partner. Kalsched (1996: 93) identifies this as an archetypal process which 'seems to involve an attack by one pole of the archetype on the other pole, i.e., an attack of the "spirit" on affect/instinct or of the mind on the body-self'. He suggests that the powerful and daimonic images are the psyche's self-portrait of its own archetypal defences. These defences are those of splitting, projective identification, idealization and other primitive, dissociative mechanisms, the clinical features of which have been most vividly described by Klein and the post-Kleinians (even though their view is that the roots of these defences lie in instinctual drives, a view that I hope I have by now convinced the reader to reject). Kalsched's (1996) view is that even the most persecutory fantasy figures fulfil a protective function, for example by fragmenting, encapsulating or numbing the vulnerable 'personal spirit', or otherwise attacking it from inside in order to preserve it from further assault from the outside world. However, he points out that the psyche has to pay a huge price for this kind of 'total defence' (Fordham 1985) in that

> once the trauma defence is organized, all relations with the outside world are 'screened' by the self-care system. What was intended to be a defense against further trauma becomes a major resistance to all unguarded spontaneous expressions of self in the world. The person survives but cannot live creatively.
>
> (Kalsched 1996: 4)

Kalsched's (1996) model is illuminating in his description of a recognizable pattern of rigid defences demonstrated by many victims of prolonged or severe trauma experienced in early life. However, this way of understanding the self-traumatizing states that seem so persistent needs further elaboration, in terms of a clearer understanding of the developmental processes that produce these primitive defences and repeatedly activate them in later life. I agree with Kalsched when he says that it is not enough to view these defences as internalization of, and identification with, the aggressor because they often seem 'far more sadistic and brutal than any outer perpetrator' (Kalsched 1996: 4).

A developmental account of archetypal defences

I think that it is possible to expand on Kalsched's account of the development of archetypal defences, rather than identifying them as aspects of the collective unconscious and the self, activated by trauma. The problem with the argument, that trauma activates innate archetypal defences, is that it is increasingly undermined by the developmental research, which I reviewed in Chapter 3, and which leads to the conclusion that such imagery is emergent rather than innate. A developmental perspective on these primitive patterns of defence needs to explain the emergence of the grandiose defences that are activated by trauma. Such an explanation would draw on two processes, the first of these being the construction of defensive internal working models in which fantasies offer some kind of meaningful links between experiences that would otherwise seem terrifyingly random and chaotic. A developmental model would also draw on the activation of the bipolar infantile internal working models that Fonagy describes, which contain images of oneself as both omnipotent and helpless.

Trauma is bound to distort the developmental formation of internal working models. Kalsched (1996) describes the mytho-poetic function of psyche, a concept akin to that of narrative competence in attachment theory (see Chapter 6). Defences are not only avoidance mechanisms, but also active constructions in the form of narratives, created in imagination and fantasy to support a positive sense of identity and personal worth when these are threatened, by cruelty, hostility or indifference from those whom we love and on whom we are most dependent. To feel that one is of no value, unlovable or the object of hatred is unbearable. Trauma of this kind results in the defensive construction of imaginative narratives, which render the child's experience of it more bearable and less threatening to the child's very identity. One aspect of these narratives is that the child feels that his or her own vulnerability, naivety and dependence were the cause of the trauma and therefore unconsciously condemns and persecutes any such weakness whenever it emerges. Whereas Kalsched (1996) describes this as the activation of archetypal defences, I would suggest that this is also partly a process of imaginative construction which serves to alert the child to the danger of entering into any relationship where the trauma might be repeated. It reflects a defensive narrative, based on the operation of an internal working model in which all vulnerability must be avoided or it will be met with abuse or punishment. These defensive fantasies then continue to form an integral part of the core internal working models, which organize the sense of self in relationship with others and with the world.

Garwood (1996) offers clinical evidence which supports this pattern of response to extreme cruelty. He draws on the terrible Holocaust experience of his own family members as well as his patients to suggest that one of the key features of this extreme form of trauma is the absolute powerlessness of the victims. He suggests:

> Self-blame and consequential guilt, though still causing great psychic pain, are emotionally less painful, anxiety provoking and overwhelming than powerlessness. They create a self-

empowering omnipotent phantasy which presupposes responsibility and the power, ability and possibility to exercise it.

(Garwood 1996: 247)

In addition, as Kalsched (1996) points out, the human being constantly searches for meaningful links but trauma reverses this
process by creating dissociative defences which fragment an
unbearable experience into parts, so that its full horror is miti-
gated. It is a powerful example of Jung's insight that an insuper-
able obstacle in the present gives rise to a retreat to infantile modes
of psychic functioning and their accompanying primitive defences.
Jung anticipated this attachment theory view of defences when he
recognized that regressive fantasy may be mobilized as a kind of
psychic protection when someone is faced with a present-day
situation which feels unbearable or seems insoluble. He understood
that infantile fantasies may function in this way rather than being
the causative agents of neurosis. Jung wrote:

> For these reasons I no longer seek the cause of a neurosis in
> the past, but in the present. I ask, what is the necessary task
> which the patient will not accomplish? The long list of his
> infantile fantasies does not give me any sufficient aetiological
> explanation because I know that these fantasies are only puffed
> up by the regressive libido, which has not found its natural
> outlet in a new form of adaptation to the demands of life.
>
> (Jung 1916: para. 570)

He also identified that these fantasies frequently take on an infantile
grandiose character, writing: 'In other cases the fantasies have more
the character of wonderful ideals which put beautiful and airy
phantasms in place of crude reality' (Jung 1913: para. 404). Jung
later increasingly recognized that this kind of defensive response
may be maladaptive and itself perpetuate the problem, in that a
present-day difficulty activates a dissociated part of the mind, a
complex, which then dominates mental functioning inappropriately
and without self-reflection.

It is striking how similar this view is to that of one of the most
distinguished contemporary psychoanalysts, Joseph Sandler, who
suggested that regression can be understood as 'the re-employment
of previous structures that have been inhibited in the course of
development' (Sandler and Joffe 1967). Fonagy elaborates:

'Normally, archaic processes remain present but hidden by more efficient ego processes. It is only in response to pathological inhibition or breakdown of the higher order processes that such obsolescent aspects become manifest' (Fonagy 1991: 653). The kind of primitive defences which are activated by trauma includes the grandiose omnipotence of early infancy, which might well be expressed in the form of magical or terrifying figures whose protective function may take the form of the attacks on the vulnerable 'personal spirit', so vividly described by Kalsched (1996). The difference is that I regard these as the activation of early developmental states and their accompanying imagery rather than viewing them as innate. In *The Inner World of Trauma*, Kalsched does not clarify his views on the origin of archetypal defences, describing one patient's archaic archetypal figure as 'personifying the terrifying dismembering rage of the collective psyche', representing the dark side of the self (Kalsched 1996: 17). This would seem to imply an innate image, somehow existing prior to experience and waiting to be activated under certain extreme conditions; I explored the internal inconsistencies of this model in Chapter 2. However, in a more recent article, Kalsched (2003) offers a clearer developmental account of archetypal defences. He uses the striking metaphor of the 'Big Bang' to suggest that, just as gravity pulled matter together until it agglomerated into stars in the earliest stages of the formation of the Universe, so in similar fashion

> we can imagine the early luminosities of a child's mind as archaic structures, part somatic, part mental which organize experience and – given 'good enough' mediation by the mother's empathy – provide the first intimations of 'meaning'. With the advent of symbolic language this process accelerates and the 'illumination' of the child's heretofore undifferentiated world, must be like the lighting up of the starry vault of heaven after a billion years of darkness.
>
> (Kalsched 2003)

This is an emergent model of archetypes, entirely compatible with the view of the archetype as image schema, which provides the scaffolding for the gradual creation of ever more complex symbolic meaning.

In addition, severe trauma may affect even these earliest stages of psychic development, that of image schema formation. I will take one example of an image schema described by Johnson (1987), that of 'links'. Johnson suggests that the 'link' schema initially reflects the infant's awareness of connection between two physical objects, but this is then metaphorically extended to make possible our perception of temporal connections, in which event A follows event B, functional linking, in which parts are related to each other as part of a functioning whole (e.g. arms and legs as part of the body) and similarity in which some abstract connection links two or more objects (Johnson 1987: 117). He does not discuss the impact of trauma on the formation of these metaphorical extensions of image schemas but I would suggest that extreme dissociative states might result from the traumatic disruption of this process. For example, in terms of the 'link' schema, a child who has never experienced the connection between the parts of his own body and that of his mother's, has never had any regular and reliable experience that feeding follows the sensation of hunger, or who has never experienced language as a safe communication, may develop very fragmented and distorted extensions of the 'link' schema, which might well appear as meaningless and terrifying, fragmented images in imagination and dreams – perhaps of the kind so well portrayed in the surrealist imagery of Salvador Dali.

This kind of information-processing account can deepen our understanding of the clinical picture that results from trauma and of the distortion of the archetypal defences that it produces. A developmental failure, or a trauma-induced disruption, of the 'link' schema would be entirely consistent with Kalsched's view that 'an "archaic defense" seems to rupture the integrated functioning of the archetype, severing the links between affect and image, thereby rendering experience meaningless' (Kalsched 1996: 93).

Dissociative and constructive aspects of defences

I hope that it will have become clear by now that defences serve a twofold purpose. On the one hand, defences serve to fragment painful meaning, rendering it less unbearable by a process of dissociation and compartmentalization. On the other hand, defences are also attempts at repair, constructing new and less distressing symbolic significance which renders trauma less threatening to one's personal sense of worth and identity. In both cases the internal working model is the key, in that the dissociative process leads in time to multiple dissociated internal working models which may be activated and alternate unpredictably, giving rise to the 'stable instability' of borderline personality disorder. Constructive processes give rise to internal working models which contain less distressing interpetations of painful realities, although as Bucci points out: '[t]he new symbols that are incorporated in the attempted repair may be adaptive or dysfunctional to varying degrees' (Bucci 1997: 205). Bucci describes this balance between the dissociative and integrative role of defences:

> Defenses may be characterized as incorporating both dissoci-ation and attempted repair, and may be distinguished in terms of their relative emphases with respect to these functions. I would suggest that defenses that are destructive of symbolic meaning are more likely to be considered low level or regres-sive; higher level defenses are those that carry some symbolic meaning of their own.
>
> (Bucci 1997: 205)

Trauma, defences and neurobiology

The impact of trauma on the brain is complex and as yet only partially understood (LeDoux 1998). Wilkinson (2003) has reviewed the available evidence relating to the development of the brain in healthy childhood and under the impact of trauma and concludes that 'whether the trauma is physical, psychological or sexual it sets off a ripple of hormonal changes that organize the brain to cope in a hostile world' (Wilkinson 2003).

It may not be possible to integrate fully an information-processing perspective which focuses on the nature and content of internal working models with a neurobiological approach which examines the impact of trauma on the structure and functioning of neuronal pathways. However, some links can be made between these two levels of explanation, in that the higher cognitive appraisal, by which we attribute meaning to experience, determines the degree of fear and anxiety aroused by implicit and explicit memories. This evaluation, itself stored in internal working models, plays a crucial role in determining the degree of stress that a person experiences in a given situation or the amount of anxiety aroused by any particular memory. LeDoux (1998) supports the view that cognition has a direct impact on neurophysiology, suggesting that the cognitions linked to emotional arousal stimulate the amygdala which in turn facilitates the cortical awareness of anxious thoughts and memories. 'The brain enters into a vicious cycle of emotional and cognitive excitement' (LeDoux 1998: 257). The extent to which strategies such as the construction of defensive fantasies is successful in diminishing the stress aroused by memories of trauma is also therefore a factor to be taken into account when exploring the impact of trauma.

The effect of stress is to stimulate the production of the hormone cortisol which, when secreted in excess, is toxic to parts of the brain such as the hypothalamus and hippocampus. Animal studies have shown that repeated high exposure to high levels of circulating stress hormones such as cortisol results in destruction of the parts of the brain that are responsive to these hormones in the bloodstream. LeDoux (1998) suggests that the resulting malfunctions in the hippocampal memory function may lead to a failure to recall details of an instigating trauma. It is therefore probably impossible to evaluate the extent to which loss of memory for traumatic events is due to one of three mechanisms:

- first, a stress-related attentional narrowing that occurs in situations arousing fear, such as any traumatic event
- second, a defensive avoidance of distressing memories of trauma, whether this is conceptualized as repression, dissociation or defensive exclusion
- third, a physiological failure of hippocampal function which cannot really be considered as a psychodynamic defence.

However, there is a final possibility which complicates the picture even further, which is that the defensive avoidance of distressing memories may in itself lead in the long term to a disuse atrophy of neurophysiological pathways – defensive avoidance may itself lead to hippocampal atrophy. Emotional regulation patterns established in early childhood may also have a lasting effect on the response of the amygdala to fear and on connections between the prefrontal cortex and the limbic system (Fonagy 2001: 46).

Another feature of trauma is the phenomenon of post-traumatic stress disorder, in which memories are not lost but, on the contrary, are activated automatically and involuntarily. LeDoux suggests that direct projections from the sub-cortical sensory systems activate the amygdala which triggers the accompanying fear reactions 'before the cortex has a chance to figure out what it is that is being reacted to' (LeDoux 1998: 257). In other words, the neurophysio-logical response is dissociated from the appraisal process rooted in the internal working models that are the manifestations of higher cortical function. However, this automatic physiological process may itself reinforce psychodynamic defences; after each occasion in which a flashback occurs, the traumatized person will identify features of the environment or of their own state of mind that may have triggered the 'flashback' and will avoid those situations or thoughts on future occasions. This is a form of repression or defensive exclusion, an avoidance of the experiences whose significance might indicate further trauma. For example, a war veteran may have flashbacks that are triggered by any sudden loud noise and may quickly learn to avoid any situation in which that is likely to happen. These defensive strategies are initially conscious but may become involuntary and unconscious over time.

Clinical illustration

A patient experienced a sudden and traumatic separation from his parents at the age of 5, when he was rushed into an isolation hospital with scarlet fever. His parents were only allowed to wave to him through a glass screen and the nurses treated him harshly, smacking him when he vigorously stirred the jam into his rice pudding. He had recently learnt to read and he remembers that he spent as much time as possible reading to avoid thinking about the painful reality of his actual situation. Later in life he continued to use reading as a way to avoid distressing experiences, particularly those around separation, but was not aware of the defensive nature of this until the pattern was pointed out to him.

Conclusion

An attachment perspective on defences highlights a two-way process in relation to the meaning and significance of experience. Defences serve both to fragment unbearable meaning and also to construct new and more acceptable narratives in imagination and fantasy. One frequent criticism of attachment theory is that it is too concerned with the effect of external events and not enough with the reality of the unconscious intrapsychic world, a criticism which I believe is based on a fundamental misconception. Attachment theory is truly a theory which integrates the intrapsychic and the interpersonal in that its primary focus is on the unconscious intra-psychic meaning of unconscious interpersonal interactions. The core theoretical concept in attachment theory is that of the internal working model and the research tools, the Strange Situation and the Adult Attachment Interview, are measures of the impact of the unconscious internal working models of key attachment figures on the adult or child subject – they are not merely measures of the impact of parental behaviour. A child's very real experience of the parental unconscious cannot be overemphasized and has been demonstrated time and again.

Finally, I shall end this discussion by pointing out that there are some people for whom all defences may fail, in the face of over-whelming and consistent mental or physical abuse, neglect or indifference. The terrifying experience of a parent's cruelty, mal-evolence or destructive intent can sometimes be defended against only by the elimination of thought itself; Shirley Wheeley (1992) captured this idea beautifully in the title of her article 'Looks that kill the capacity for thought', and this leads me on to another key concept in attachment theory, that of reflective function, which is the capacity to be aware of oneself and others as independent psychological and emotional beings. The abandonment of this crucial awareness may be the last and most extreme dissociative defence of those faced with intolerable cruelty in others. Michael Fordham described a similar extreme defence, for which he coined the phrase 'defences of the self' (Fordham 1985[1947]: 152). I shall explore these ultimate defences further in Chapter 6.

Reflective function

The mind as an internal object

In the previous chapters I have described the reconceptualization of the internal world that Bowlby initiated, which has been developed by subsequent attachment theorists. I have indicated some of the issues which opened up when Bowlby started to question the psychoanalytic view of the nature and formation of internal objects and introduced the idea of the internal working model with internalization as the key to the formation of unconscious patterns or structures in the psyche. His insistence on the powerful effect of external reality on the infant psyche and his view that the internalization of that reality was the key process in the formation of the unconscious internal world eventually led to his alienation from the psychoanalytic community, a fracture which is only now beginning to be healed (Eagle 1995; Holmes 2001).

One of the most important features of the internal working model is the fact that it represents the repeated patterns of relationship with key attachment figures. These patterns are represented in the form of implicit rules, beliefs and expectations about the behaviour and attitudes of the caregiver, as I described in Chapter 4. Internal working models of key attachment figures are therefore rooted in real experience that begin to develop in the first year of an infant's life; they incorporate considerable information about the parents, not only in terms of their behaviour but also about their mental and emotional lives. A child's tendency to 'incorporate mental state attributions into internal working models of self–other relationships depends on the opportunities that he had in early life to observe and explore the mind of his primary caregiver' (Fonagy 2001: 167).

The concept of reflective function

How do we become aware that other people are not just 'objects' but reflecting beings with thoughts, beliefs, judgements, desires, intentions, everything that goes to make up the human mental and emotional world? How do we also become aware of ourselves as psychological agents, whose mental processes produce an effect on and so create a response in people around us?

This capacity is called 'reflective function', a term which seems preferable to 'metacognitive monitoring', 'mind-mindedness' or 'mentalization', all of which have also been used to describe the awareness of oneself and others as psychological and emotional beings as well as physical objects. Reflective function depends upon the creation of adequate internal working models of mental functioning in all its aspects, including emotions, intentions and desires as well as thoughts; one might say that reflective function requires the construction of internal working models of internal working models. Mary Main's research with the Adult Attachment Interview (Main and Goldwyn 1995) has shown that reflective function underpins the capacity to give a coherent and reflective account of one's own life. Reflective function can be measured (Fonagy 1995: 250-1). It is the most significant and compelling evidence of adult security and the most predictive of infant security; reflective function demonstrates that a person has formed internally consistent working models of relationships in which the behaviour of key attachment figures can be experienced as an empathic response to the infant's needs, and so, consistent, meaningful and containing.

People who have failed to develop reflective function treat themselves and others as merely physical objects and lack the capacity to empathize with other people or to place their own emotions in a meaningful context, to reflect on them and so experience them in a safe way. As parents, such people will therefore also fail to respond in a reflective and empathic way to an infant's distress and so fail to make him or her feel understood and safe. In this chapter I will explore the effect of this failure of reflective function on the child's psychological development and the specific clinical features that result.

Theory of mind

What are the developmental processes which underpin the development of reflective function? Empirical research in this area has focused on the concept of 'theory of mind', which is the growing child's capacity to be aware that other people have different ideas and beliefs from his or her own. This seems to be the first step towards a growing awareness that people are mentally as well as physically separate. The classic experiment to demonstrate this involves showing small children a cardboard 'Smarties' tube and asking them what they thought it contained. As expected, they all replied 'Smarties'. The lid was then removed and the children saw that the tube contained a pencil. The tube was then closed again and each child was asked what the tube contained and then what their friend, who was waiting outside, would think was in the tube. All the 3 year olds were able to say correctly that the tube contained a pencil, but then said that they thought their friend, who had not seen the tube contents, would also think that it contained a pencil. The 4 year olds, on the other hand, could correctly anticipate that their friend outside would expect 'Smarties' in the tube; they could understand that another person would have a different belief from their own (Perner *et al.* 1987).

This ability to take account of states of mind in predicting how other people will behave is one of the capacities which defines the human mind. This 'theory of mind' allows us to understand psychological cause and effect and so to anticipate correctly another person's attitudes; it is therefore probably at least as important an effective skill, as a mechanism for survival in evolutionary terms, as understanding physical cause and effect. Babies survive the long period of helplessness in infancy through the relationship with their parents, and this relationship is rooted in the intense resonance of mutual reflectiveness between parent and baby. How can natural selection have brought this about? The intensity of relationship itself is not, indeed could not, be genetically encoded for the reasons I have explored in Chapter 3. Genes simply do not encode emotional and cognitive information of that kind. Instead, simple hard-wired genetic mechanisms, such as 'Conspec' (see Chapter 3), which maximize the attention that a newborn baby gives to any human face which appears in the infant's visual field, provide a necessary foundation on which further developmental processes can then be built.

The attachment system itself is one such 'emergent' pattern, which is reliably constructed in the repeated interactions between mother and baby. Some of the key building blocks in this emergent process are beginning to become clear. For example, Fonagy (2001) explores in more detail the survival value that an infant's expressions of distress may have, pointing out that high stress levels in response to possible danger risks the creation of developmental abnormalities due to high circulating levels of cortisol. Attracting protective responses from the caregiver could have developed in less stressful ways. However, Fonagy offers a more subtle explanation for the survival value of the infant's distress:

> The infant's distress not only brings the caregiver physically close to the child but also creates comparable distress in the object. Thus an ideal situation is created for the infant to experience containment (Bion 1962), accurate mirroring (Winnicott 1971[1967]), in other words, a context within which internalization processes essential to self-development can take place. The evolutionary function of the attachment system thus may not be the eliciting of a protective response from a human adult, as Bowlby thought. Rather the survival risks to the organism entailed in the processes of attachment are justified by the benefit that the experience of psychic containment brings in terms of the development of a coherent and symbolizing self.
>
> (Fonagy 2001: 187)

Fonagy has thus clarified the concept of mirroring by suggesting that it is not only the image of the emotionally containing parent which is internalized. For reflective function to develop, the infant also has to internalize the parent as someone with a mental image of the infant, a parent who sees the infant as someone with a mind and emotions. It is the parent's mental representation of the infant which is internalized, allowing the infant to find him- or herself in the other. If the parent fails in this respect, the version of itself that the infant encounters in the parent's mind is that of a physical object rather than a person with a mind of his or her own. Under these circumstances, it is difficult to see how infants could experience themselves as a reflective beings.

In addition, Gergely and Watson (1996) have spelt out some of the key features of the parents' responses that help the infant to develop a gradual awareness of his or her own emotions and states of mind. They have shown that the concept of mirroring needs radical revision, in that parents who are highly attuned to their baby's emotional state do not merely copy the infant's emotional expressions but instead produce a markedly exaggerated response and playful 'pretend' response. Gergely and Watson (1996) suggest that this 'marked' response enables the infant to identify the response as a reflection of the infant's own emotions, whereas parents' normal 'unmarked' emotional expressions are not interpreted as reflections of the infant's own emotional world.

There is empirical evidence which supports this conceptual model, showing that reflective function seems to develop only in a reasonably secure attachment and that it depends on the parents' reflective capacity for events to link in a meaningful way for the baby. Fonagy's research has shown that mothers who were highly stressed and deprived in terms of numerous social and economic factors nevertheless had securely attached children if they themselves had high ratings on a scale measuring reflective function, whereas mothers who scored low on reflective function had children who showed insecure attachment (Fonagy 1995).

Reflective function as the root of our sense of meaning and capacity to symbolize

It begins to become clear that the concept of reflective function has enormous implications for our understanding of human psychological development and functioning and in particular for the development of a sense of meaning – a word that we all intuitively understand but which a moment's reflection shows us to be rather vague and imprecise. What are the contributing factors to a sense of meaning, which is rooted in the capacity to find symbolic significance in our experience?

I would suggest that there are four key and interrelated elements, all of which contribute to the development of reflective function:

- *narrative competence:* the recognition of psychological cause and effect, which links events in a meaningful way and is the basis for a sense of agency
- *intentionality:* the capacity to pursue goals and desires, that is, to have a mental appetite

- *appraisal:* the capacity to evaluate the relative significance of experiences
- *individuation:* the awareness of one's own and other people's independent subjectivity.

Developmental considerations

I intend to show that these are interrelated aspects of reflective function, whose essence is the capacity to experience one's own and other people's psychological separateness and individuality. Theory of mind is the necessary foundation stone for reflective function, in that it involves the awareness that other people have different thoughts and beliefs from one's own. However, reflective function is much more than this, in that it extends the awareness of psychological separateness to include the knowledge that other people have different emotions, desires and intentions as well. It also extends the awareness of psychological individuality into the recognition of the emotional and intentional world of the other, beyond the cognitive level demonstrated in the 'Smarties' experiment.

Empirical research increasingly suggests that theory of mind is not a one-off achievement but a gradually evolving capacity that becomes increasingly sophisticated and complex. As Gergely *et al.* (1995: 166) state: 'There is also a growing body of evidence concerning the developmental unfolding of the child's naïve theory of mind between the second and fifth year'. I would suggest that there is a spectrum with the simplest cognitive aspects of 'theory of mind' at one end and the full expression of reflective function at the other. Perhaps the latter is fully achieved by only a small proportion of people in the course of a lifetime. The concepts I have chosen to explore as aspects of reflective function are those that have been demonstrated empirically to be manifestations of theory of mind in small children, and which also develop into more sophisticated and complex abilities with the growth and development of reflective function throughout life.

For example, Gergely *et al.* (1995) have carefully studied the development of the 'intentional stance' in small children, showing that the capacity to attribute mental intentions to another person emerges in its earliest and most simple form at about the age of 12 months. Understanding the other person's intentions then allows the child to predict and explain their behaviour, a crucial developmental achievement and a central feature of theory of mind. However, it is easy to deduce that if an understanding of the other's intentions gives rise to fear and distress, then the understanding of intentionality itself may become the focus for defensive exclusion. This may include a person's awareness of their own intentions and so of their own desires, if these are themselves likely to cause distress, for example by bringing that person into conflict with others. This is explored in more detail later.

Similarly, Jean Mandler (1988) has shown that appraisal is a key aspect of the development of theory of mind. She argues that the capacity to form meaningful concepts depends upon a very specific form of appraisal, perceptual analysis, that develops from about 6 months onwards. Perceptual analysis is 'a symbolic process by which one perception is actively compared with another' and this appraisal process is the first building block of conceptual thought (Mandler 1988: 126). However, like the 'intentional stance', appraisal develops into a much more complex ability throughout development. Kobak (1999: 28) points out that appraisal lies at the heart of separation distress; for example, if physical proximity to the parent is the key to separation anxiety, then infants should respond with the same level of alarm to separations regardless of the circumstances. However, the Strange Situation demonstrates that infants show more distress on separations in an unfamiliar environment than at home and also on a second separation than on the first. These findings can be explained by viewing the infant's distress 'as resulting from the child's appraisal or evaluation of the mother's departure, and not from the actual physical absence of the parent' (Kobak 1999: 28). Similarly, the variations in the infant's behaviour in response to reunion result from the different expectations of how their mothers will respond to them, and of their mothers' availability to them.

Mahler's (1975) work on separation–individuation has highlighted the fact that it is the intrapsychic achievement of a sense of separateness from mother which gradually leads to clear intrapsychic representations of the self as distinguished from representations of the object world and so to the child's sense of being a separate individual (Mahler 1975: 8). This process seems to be highly dependent on the parent's capacity to reflect on, and so modulate, the mental states which underlie her baby's behaviour and communications. Fonagy (2001: 172) suggests that children who have not received recognizable but modified images of their affective states, through their parents' responses to them, may have trouble in differentiating physical from psychic reality. This failure to develop internal representations of mind (the mind as an internal object or internal working model) underlies the failure to develop a sense of psychological separateness; in this situation emotions are not used or experienced as communications but as manipulations, which make other people do things rather than conveying one's own mental state to them to respond to as they choose.

The failure of reflective function

The concept of reflective function can cast a new light on a whole range of the problems that our patients present us with in the consulting room particularly, as I have already indicated, those in which a person's behaviour seems mindless, in that it seems disconnected from any sense of judgement, intention, desire or relatedness to others. Under these circumstances, the world and life itself are meaningless. Reflective function can help us gain a better understanding of many symptoms or patterns, which otherwise can seem rather non-specific and difficult to identify and can also give us a new interpretative tool for working with patients who have familiar clinical patterns of psychological disturbance that are very resistant to change in analysis.

A distinction needs to be made between failure of reflective function as a developmental deficit and the avoidance of reflective function as an unconscious defence against psychological distress. In the former case, the capacity for the most elementary theory of mind does not seem to develop at all and it has been suggested that this is the crucial factor in the development of autism (Baron-Cohen 1988). In the latter case the inhibition of reflective function is partial and consists of a defensive avoidance of the awareness of mental and emotional states in oneself and others. This defensive failure of reflective function not only may play a part in specific clinical syndromes (in ways that I shall explore later), but also is apparent in certain unconscious defences which we see in many of our more disturbed patients, regardless of their presenting problems. In my experience the interpretation of these defences as an unconscious avoidance of reflective function has often been the most effective way to overcome the kind of impasse which is reached when the patient resists any attempt on the analyst's part to find meaning in the patient's behaviour or communications.

I shall therefore also explore here the consequences of the defensive exclusion of key processes such as narrative competence, intentionality and appraisal, which contribute to reflective capacity. Fonagy (1991) has shown that many characteristics of borderline states can be understood as a defensive avoidance of reflective function, but he has not examined the clinical patterns that may result from defensive exclusion of each of these specific components of reflective function. Cortina (2003) has explained how such a defensive exclusion might arise. He takes up Bowlby's observation that information that is perceived as potentially dangerous activates defensive strategies such as compartmentalization, filtering or perceptual blocking, leading to defensive exclusion. These defensive processes were discussed in detail in Chapter 5. Cortina further proposes that emotions act as 'psycho-physiological markers that alert the organism to important information coming from within the organism or the environment'. If reflective function itself has come to be perceived as a threat, then emotion may act as a signal that the meaning-making process itself must be avoided; I hope to illustrate this more clearly with the examples I give below.

Narrative competence: the recognition of psychological cause and effect

It is psychological links that give stories their meaning. One of the defining features of any narrative is that it links events in a meaningful way through the desires and intentions of the people who play the various roles in the story, whether fictional or not. In any narrative it is minds which are the agents of change, giving rise to decisions, choices and actions which produce effects and which link events into a coherent structure. Without mental agency, there would be no story, no meaningful thread tying events together and those events would appear random and meaningless.

This capacity of reflective function to link experiences in a meaningful way is a crucial part of human psychological development and is intuitively nurtured by parents in the early development of their children as much, for example, as the nurturing of language itself. One of the key functions of stories is to facilitate the child's understanding of this link between what goes on in people's minds and the practical consequences, a process that developmental psychologists have come to recognize as vital. Stories allow a child to explore the possibilities for future events and so to investigate how the choices that people make influence events (Bruner 1986; Emde 1999).

Holmes (2001) has coined the term 'narrative competence' to describe this ability to make sense of experiences and has investigated a range of deficits in the development of narrative capacity, linking these with differing patterns of insecure attachment. In secure attachment, there is a coherence in the overall narrative and the teller of the story is neither detached and dissociated, nor overwhelmed by undifferentiated emotion. In contrast, insecure attachment is characterized in ambivalent patients by stories that are over-elaborated and enmeshed and in avoidant patients by accounts that are dismissive and lacking in meaningful detail (Holmes 2001: 86). A parent who is unable to tune his or her understanding to the child's may impede the development of this aspect of reflective function.

CLINICAL ILLUSTRATION

A patient dreamt that he was taking a history exam but he could not understand any of the questions and started to suffer from an intense headache; he left the exam but returned on another occasion for a second attempt. This time the crippling headache started as he was walking up the stairs towards the examination room. The examiner, a friend of his father's, expressed severe disappointment in him and had expected him to do better.

It seemed to me that this dream demonstrated how difficult my patient found it to make meaningful sense of his own history (taking a history exam) and how painful this lack of narrative competence was for him, an awareness conveyed in the dream image of a headache. His parents had been unable to see the vital importance of imaginative play and had treated him as though they expected him to be a small adult and these unrealistic expectations had blocked the development of narrative competence.

THE 'NARRATIVE DIALOGUE'

Holmes also highlights the fact that narrative is a dialogue: 'There is always another to whom the Self is telling his or her story, even if in adults this takes the form of an internal dialogue' (Holmes 2001:

85). This dialogue is also itself a constructive process of increasing complexity in which a story is created first by one person and is then taken over and retold on a new level by the other. This 'narrative dialogue' continues throughout development, from the earliest moments of an infant's life, and plays a central role in psychotherapeutic dialogue. Bion's (1962) concept of 'reverie' describes the mother's role in creating a narrative that she can use to give meaning to her infant's various behaviours, interpreting them as meaningful communications. At this stage the mother holds the storyline and the infant gradually internalizes the meaningful links that she has made for him or her. In this way infants gradually acquire the awareness of their own mind with its feelings and thoughts and the sense of their mind as an agent of change, because when they want something, his mother produces it.

However, in early childhood, the role of narrative changes, as the magical nature of mental functioning is explored. Small children need fairy tales to be repeated over and over again and avidly absorb their meaning for themselves. For example, in the story of *Cinderella*, her desire to go to the ball is magically translated into physical reality by her fairy godmother's goodwill towards her, just as mothers, through their own reflective function, can understand what is in their babies' minds and, in producing the desired object, magically transforms the baby's wishes into reality. At this stage narratives, in the form of magical fairy tales, give a language to the stage of narcissistic omnipotence and grandiosity that is crucial as the foundation for a secure sense of self and self-esteem. These infantile fantasies of grandiosity serve a crucial role as defences against too intense an awareness of the child's helplessness and vulnerability.

However, narrative is also the vehicle for the process of disillusionment which is vital for a child to appreciate his or her real limitations and so for a healthy narcissism to emerge that is not based on omnipotence and that can survive disappointment and failure (Winnicott 1971: 11). Once again, fairy tales can play a vital part in this process, in teaching children about other, apparently less desirable consequences of wishes and intentions, showing that their own minds can have a powerful effect and that their own choices and attitudes have consequences for other people. In the story of *The Princess and the Frog*, the princess makes a promise to the frog that she will love him and let him live with her if he rescues her favourite golden ball from the bottom of the pond where it has fallen. However, once the frog has retrieved the ball, the princess runs off and forgets her promise to him. She has not yet learnt that her promise has been taken by the frog to be a true reflection of her intentions and that her mental processes mattered to him. The frog expected her to take his wishes seriously. The frog's reappearance in her home and her father's insistence that she keeps her promise force her to face the reality of the effect of her own psychological processes on other people. The final turn to the story is that once she does so, the frog can become fully human, so that her reflective function has a magical redemptive effect.

This process whereby the narrative initially belongs to the parent and then is taken over by the child is also mirrored in the analytic dialogue. Our analytic theories are narratives that we construct so that we can provide an analytic reverie which allows us to find meaning in our patients' verbal and non-verbal communications when the patients themselves cannot yet do so. A successful analytic narrative is one that can become meaningful to our patients so that they can take it over, use it for themselves and adapt it to establish their own sense of psychic causality, of the link between intrapsychic experiences and the external world. Holmes (2001) describes the psychotherapist's role in this respect as that of an 'assistant autobiographer', whose role is to find stories that correspond to experience. This role starts in the assessment interview, where the therapist will 'use her narrative competence to help the patient shape the story into a more coherent pattern'. He suggests that the patient then gradually

> learns to build up a 'story-telling function', which takes experience from 'below' and, in the light of overall meanings 'from above' (which can be seen as themselves stored or condensed stories) supplied by the therapist, fashions a new narrative about her self and her world.
>
> (Holmes 2001: 85)

This constructive aspect of analytic work is explored in more detail in Chapter 7.

Intentionality: the capacity to pursue goals and desires

The concept of reflective function is the foundation stone of the capacity for intentions; intentions, in turn, form the basis for desires and appetites. There are many people who simply do not seem to know what they want, what interests them or excites their attention. They seem trapped in a passive prison in which they are doomed to respond endlessly to other people's demands on them, because the alternative is a terrifying emptiness and aimlessness born out of the absence of desire.

There is a vital distinction to be made here between an appetite on the one hand and greed on the other. An appetite of any kind, symbolic or physical, is directed towards a specific object and can be satisfied after a certain enjoyment of that object. Greed, however, is often indiscriminate, insatiable and gives no real pleasure – consumption is not an enjoyable experience.

The concept of reflective function can help us understand this distinction between an appetite and greed. Appetite requires a mind which knows what it wants, how much and when it has had enough; all these are aspects of intentionality and the sense of purpose and direction required in order to be able to desire, relate to and enjoy the object. Greed, on the other hand, is conspicuous by the absence of any such evidence of reflective function at work, the lack of any discrimination in relation to the quality of an experience. A person in the grip of greed of any kind seems, and often feels, 'mindless'; this can be helpful in thinking about certain clinical patterns in which the person's behaviour seems mindless in the sense that it is apparently disconnected from any sense of intention or desire. It seems to be particularly relevant to the understanding of eating disorders, particularly bulimia where binge-eating seems to provide a mechanism for patients to eliminate temporarily any sense of themselves as an intentional agent; the link between mind and behaviour is broken, in that individuals may not consciously wish to binge, but nevertheless observe themselves buying and eating the food. A mindless, joyless greed replaces appetite or desire and the absence of reflective function prevents any further evaluation of this behaviour. The person has no sense of his or her own mind at work, making decisions or choices, and the behaviour is experienced as automatic and even alien.

CLINICAL ILLUSTRATIONS

Two clinical vignettes will help to illustrate the failure of this aspect of reflective function:

The first concerns a bulimic patient whose parents seem to have had absolutely no capacity at all to relate to their children with even a minimal degree of empathy. They would become angry with the children at the slightest provocation, for example, hitting them if they cried. My patient's attachment needs went entirely unrecognized and were treated as physical demands, for example, for food. It seems to have been an utterly confusing and at times terrifying world for my patient, in which she never felt understood, loved or cared for. Her emotions were a mystery to her just as they were to her parents, who seem to have lacked all reflective capacity.

As an adult my patient has a lack of reflective capacity herself, in that she seems unable to be aware of and evaluate the meaning of her own reactions and emotions. It is as though she cannot use her own judgement at all to make sense of her own experience of the world around her. She remains entirely dependent on me to understand the meaning of the events she describes and to explain her own reactions to her so that they can acquire psychological meaning. Any misunderstanding on my part feels catastrophic to her; she often says that she wants me to make things better for her and that if I don't say exactly the right thing, it must be because I don't care and don't want to help her. I should know exactly what is in her mind without her having to tell me and if I fail, she then experiences me as hostile and malevolent, just as she felt her parents were. This is an intolerable state of mind for her and she has found that binge-eating seems to be a successful way to get rid of this painful state because when she is bingeing her mind becomes empty. She temporarily succeeds in making herself mindless and eliminating any awareness of mental processes, both in herself and in the person who has hurt her.

The same patient has also described a defensive use of eating patterns in relation to anorexic episodes which she goes through from time to time. She discovered in her early teens that chronic restriction of her food intake would lead to semi-starvation. She found that she could regulate this in order to maintain a state of mind which she describes as 'spaced out', where tiredness and a feeling of light-headedness produced a mildly dissociated state, in which nothing matters to her very much and she remains detached from and unaffected by people around her. In this state of mind she is protected from the distress that she often otherwise feels people can so easily cause her by any lack of empathy on their part towards her, because she no longer cares about them or about herself. She has learnt to control her food intake quite precisely in order to maintain this dissociated state while not starving herself to the point where she becomes physically ill. Anorexia has become a mechanism for eliminating reflective function.

A second patient suffers from intermittent episodes of bulimia, usually associated with a mood of angry depression and an attitude of loathing and contempt for herself. At these times she feels that she is a bad person and that everything she does is rubbish. She cannot usually identify any reason for these feelings when she is in this state of mind but at the same time she can do nothing to change it.

During the course of the therapy it has become apparent that these states usually occur when she is actually or potentially in conflict with someone. When she feels hostile to someone she feels that she is bad because she should never be critical of others and should not pursue her own needs or desires if another person does not wish her to. She has come to recognize that the word 'bad' has become equated for her with having a mind of her own, with her own needs and desires. She was brought up by a strictly religious mother who always taught her children to put other people first and who spent hours tirelessly and selflessly doing charitable work. At the same time she seems to have been depressed and unable to enjoy being with her children so that they came to feel they could easily be a burden to her if they needed anything from her. My patient felt that her mother wanted a well-behaved doll rather than a real child with an appetite and desires of her own.

Her bulimia seems to be, at least in part, a diversionary activity whose unconscious purpose is to make herself mindless and so block out all the painful thoughts that she is a bad person.

Both of these clinical examples illustrate the defensive purpose of the elimination of intentionality by these patients. If they experience themselves and others as mindless, they do not have to be aware of hostility, malevolence or the indifference of other people towards them and their emotions, nor of their own fundamental needs for love and understanding. Sometimes being mindful can simply be too painful and it becomes preferable to eliminate all awareness of other people's minds and intentions, as well as all awareness of one's needs if they can never be met. Support for this view of eating disorders comes from research by Cole-Detke and Kobak (1996). They suggest that women with eating disorders do not have the ability to examine their own psychological states and cope instead by diverting distress to a focus on their bodies. Eating disorders thus allow the diversion of attention away from attachment-related concerns and feelings of distress and hence the avoidance of reflective function. It utilizes the mechanism of defensive exclusion described in Chapter 5.

In addition, there is often no capacity to sort experiences into a hierarchy, to decide which matter more than others and this overlaps considerably with the issue of appraisal as a manifestation of reflective function. However, it is worth distinguishing between intentionality and appraisal in that appraisal probably encapsulates the more cognitive aspects of the spectrum of reflective function, while intentionality and desire are more emotional experiences.

Appraisal: the capacity to evaluate the relative significance of experiences

Reflective function not only is the awareness of other people as mental and emotional beings, but also enables the knowledge of oneself as a person with a mind and emotions with the ability to evaluate, to make judgements about the quality and meaning of experiences. The development of reflective function depends upon the existence in a person's mind of internal working models which contain information about mental and emotional processes in oneself and others. Appraisal may be a conscious process but, in so far as it arises from the meanings stored in internal working models, it is an implicit process, operating automatically and in a form inaccessible to conscious awareness. This process of evaluating the importance of events provides an unconscious basis for a sense of psychological identity; without it, people do not feel that they have minds of their own, but always defer to other people's judgements because these feel more real than their own.

The appraisal aspect of reflective function can help us to understand certain patterns of symptoms which seem to indicate a failure of appraisal, for example, 'writing block' in which a person becomes unable to produce written work, however high the stakes may be. One such patient has blighted his academic career by ten years of failure to produce a single piece of writing. It seems as though he simply does not have an internal model of his own mind as an agent that can evaluate and select what to include or exclude in a piece of written work. Without such a model of his own mind as an agent of choice, this patient simply cannot decide how to prioritize the material at his disposal and he ends up swamped with a mass of words, phrases and sentences which torment him until he gives up in despair. A related picture is that of a person who cannot hold anything in mind, largely because he does not relate to a model of his mind as a psychic space in which information can be appraised, evaluated and given significance. All information therefore has to be stored externally, usually on pieces of paper which pile up from floor to ceiling; none of this can be taken in, evaluated and given an order of priority, so that it can be used internally.

The experience of appraisal by other people can be a source of distress and so lead to a defensive avoidance of reflective function. It does seem as though the suffering of knowing one's own mind, while still feeling that one is treated like a mindless object by others, is greater than the suffering of physical pain. Patients who frequently cut or burn themselves or take repeated small overdoses sometimes acknowledge that physical pain is more endurable than the mental pain of having a mind with thoughts, beliefs, desires and intentions, when these are treated as worthless by others. Self-harm often seems to be a defensive diversion from facing the full implications of rejection or abuse by another and the sense of personal worthlessness that this creates. Such patients often describe themselves as bad, disgusting or dirty. Interpretations in terms of identification with bad internal objects are not effective because they merely confirm to the patient that he or she has been judged as someone with something bad and destructive inside him or her. I have found that some progress can be made by pointing out the patients' unconscious fantasy that to be independent minded, to have a mind of one's own, is what they believe make them bad, disgusting or dirty in the eyes of their parent. They feel they can be lovable and valuable only when they are totally attuned to the needs of the attachment figure, a kind of 'reverse parenting' which may result from the parent's inability to tolerate his or her child's critical evaluation and independent judgement of them. A parent who dreads the child's appraisal is internalized, so that the child comes to believe that he or she is bad and dangerous whenever they think for themselves.

CLINICAL ILLUSTRATION

A patient dreamt that he was riding slowly on a bicycle behind a horse and carriage. The carriage contained a terrifying and dangerous person inside, who had no face. My patient knew this although he was not under any circumstances to look at the person or there would be disastrous consequences. There was a soldier sitting facing backwards on the back of the carriage and he was preventing everyone from getting past. Eventually he signalled his permission for my patient to pass, but the driver speeded up and my patient ended up behind again, feeling utterly frustrated.

I think that the person in the carriage represented the mindless, identity-less state that my patient sometimes falls into and which he finds terrifying. He does not know who he is or what he wants. A healthier child part of him tries to bypass this dreadful experience without looking at it but his defences (the soldier) will not permit him to leave it behind so easily.

Repeated physical trauma that arises from treatment for serious and chronic physical illness may also lead to deep shame at feeling that one is related to as primarily a physical object by others and that one's psychic world does not count. Don Kalsched raised this issue at a *Journal of Analytical Psychology* conference in Prague when responding to Gustav Bovensiepen's (2002) account of his work with such a traumatized patient; he identified

the deep shame that the trauma victim feels as the 'object' of another's subjectivity. Here is a boy whose physical condition has 'objectified' him in many painful ways. His whole first year was mostly in hospital with many intestinal operations. His mother then had to invade his body, sticking pins into his anus etc. We can only imagine the inevitable sense of alienation, the sense of being a flawed, damaged and inferior being that Tom would have grown up with. All this would have conspired to define Tom's life as an object – the object first of others' neglect or ridicule, the object second of his own 'totalitarian introject', the daimonic 'objectifier' in the psyche's archetypal defenses.

(Kalsched 2002: 262)

Individuation: the awareness of one's own and other people's independent subjectivity

The difficulty in linking events into a meaningful narrative, in having an appetite and in appraising the emotional significance of experience is often accompanied by the absence of any real sense of separateness. There is no sense of a psychic space between people, but instead an experience of being totally under the control of, or of totally controlling another person. There is no model of two separate people, each of whom can choose how to respond to the other's words and actions. At the start of this chapter I indicated that this may have its roots in a developmental deficit of reflective function, but that it may also emerge as a defensive process, as an attempt to eliminate reflective function and hence the awareness of intolerable mental states in oneself or others. In analysis this has profound effects on the therapy and on the therapist, because words are treated as controlling actions, not as symbolic communications. The therapist in this situation feels totally paralysed with no space to think for him- or herself; anything the therapist says to the patient can feel like a hostile attack which invades and forces certain responses from him or her, and the same experience is often true for the analyst. The absence of reflective function seems to lie at the root of these experiences of projective identification in that the other person is not related to as a separate person with a mind of their own.

CLINICAL ILLUSTRATION

A vivid illustration of this came from a patient's dream in which she saw a child in an underwater pool. The child was completely gripped by the tentacles of an octopus but was still breathing. The child's mother came with some poison because she knew that the only way to free the child was to give her poison which would pass through and kill the octopus. The impasse in the dream was clear: interpretations were poison that would kill the child at the same time as freeing her.

Separateness, the freedom to have a mind of one's own with its own thoughts, desires and judgements, is itself perceived as deadly.

The fear of psychic separateness, of having a mind of one's own, can lead to patterns of destructive enactment which seem to defy all kinds of interpretations, so that the analyst reaches a position of bewilderment, anger and even despair. This impasse results from patients' defensive exclusion of an awareness of their own mind – they cannot make use of symbolic interpretations because they are communications to a mind that they do not want to exist. In this situation, interpretations are experienced as coercive attempts to force an awareness of reflective function, and this may lead to an escalating resistance to such awareness. There is usually an extremely contradictory and confusing quality to analytic work with such a patient, who both denigrates and mercilessly attacks the analyst, while at the same time suggesting 'that his whole life depends upon the continuation of the analysis and its successful outcome' (Fordham 1985[1947]: 154). Fordham's description of this kind of analytic encounter, in which defences of the self are activated is particularly vivid:

In its more dramatic forms the syndrome can develop so that the interview becomes filled with negative affects and confusion, until the whole of the dialectic seems to break down. The time may be filled with denigrating the analyst's interventions, ending up in loud groans, screams or tears whenever the analyst speaks: the patient seems to use every means at his disposal to prevent the analyst's interventions from becoming meaningful, or alternatively or concurrently a meaning is given to them that is so distorted as to create confusion if not identified. Almost everything is reversed, turned upside down or subtly distorted so that direct communication becomes impossible.

(Fordham 1985[1947]: 154)

Wilkinson (2003) has clarified some aspects of the roots of this pattern in terms of the young self which can define itself only by identification rather than a true sense of identity. She describes certain traumatized adults and suggests that:

Each had a mother who tended to project her own split off, bad aspects of herself into her child. For each child to separate from mother led inexorably to abuse, but to remain at one with mother, on mother's terms, resulted in the development of a very particular kind of false or 'as if' self, which I have termed a 'cloned self', for this is what each mother really required of her child. It seems to have been this cloning of the negative that made the abuse possible; for each mother it was an attack on her own hated self in the cloned other.

(Wilkinson 2003)

The concept of reflective function can add to our understanding of these patterns, which are usually seen as manifestations of projective identification or, in Fordham's (1985[1947]) terminology, as 'defences of the self'. Projective identification as the unconscious forcible evacuation of an unbearable state of mind into the object is more fully rooted in interpersonal experience when seen in attachment theory terms. Fonagy (2001) suggests that children who are traumatized by markedly confusing, inconsistent or hostile caregiving cannot integrate the internalized images of the caregiver into a coherent pattern of self–other relationship and self-structure. Projective identification is the process whereby they evacuate these 'alien' representations into others, in order to preserve a coherent sense of self. However, in this model the unbearable mental contents do not arise from the child's own instinctual drives, but from the internalization of the parent's mind which threatens to annihilate the child's sense of separate identity from within. The same may be true in reverse, in that a child who senses that the parent cannot tolerate any psychological separateness will attempt to create a state of mental fusion by projective identification as a means of communication. In analysis, the analyst's attempts to think for him- or herself will be resisted by such a patient, who can relate only through identification and fusion and who therefore finds the analyst's reflective function intolerable. Fordham's account of defences of the self can also be seen as an avoidance of reflective function, both in the patient's own mind and in relation to the analyst's mind. The unconscious purpose is to create an analyst–patient amalgam and to destroy the analyst's creative capacities, so that the analyst is in danger of losing the 'inner real feeling of self in relation to the patient', or, in other words, of losing his or her reflective function.

'Borderline' personality

There is one clinical picture that patients present to us, which can be much more clearly understood if we think of it as a defensive failure of all the components of reflective function I have just described. Borderline personality disorder is stated in DSM-IV to affect 2 per cent of the general population and 20 per cent of psychiatric inpatients (American Psychiatric Association 1994), although British authors regard this as too high a figure and suggest that borderline personality disorder is in danger of being used indiscriminately as a synonym for personality disorder (Freeman 1994).

As defined in DSM-IV, the central features are

- impulsivity
- affective instability
- unstable self-image, aims and preferences
- chronic feelings of emptiness
- tendency to become involved in intense and unstable relationships
- efforts to avoid real or imagined abandonment
- self-destructive acts or threats are common, often in response to a fear of abandonment
- transient psychotic like episodes or dissociative states may occur in response to stress.

Many of the features of so-called borderline personality disorder can be understood as a consequence of a failure of reflective function in all its aspects, namely narrative competence, appraisal, intentionality and separation/individuation. Fonagy (1991) offers new ways of thinking about concepts such as projective identification and other pathological organizations shown in borderline functioning, relating these to the patients' difficulty in taking account of their own and others' mental states as the basis for understanding and predicting behaviour. This is the

> collection of intuitive ideas which all of us possess concerning mental functioning and the nature of perceptual experience, memory, beliefs, attributions, intentions, emotions and desires. Understanding and correctly anticipating the other's expectations and ideas is far more important than appreciating the

physical circumstances and mechanical aspects of human interaction.

(Fonagy 1991: 640)

The reflective capacity to attribute beliefs, intentions and desires to
another person becomes fully developed at about 6 years of age,
but Fonagy *et al.* (1995) suggest that this process depends upon the
availability of parent figures who themselves have this capacity to
empathize with and imagine what might be going on in the child's
mind (Fonagy *et al.* 1995). Such parents are able to respond to a
child's intentions and wishes, recognizing that the child's behaviour
reflects and communicates these. Through this process the child
comes to understand that intentions and wishes are causal in the
particular sense that they have an emotional impact on another
person and thus that they are real. Parents whose own reflective
capacity is impaired will not respond appropriately to the child's
communications and do not provide the reflective interpersonal
experiences the child needs to develop an understanding of his own
mental states.

There may also be a defensive denial of an awareness of the
thoughts and feelings of others in children who have been subject
to emotional, physical or sexual trauma. Fonagy (1991) suggests
that the development of a theory of mind depends upon a growing
awareness of the mental state of one's primary attachment figures
and that it is therefore essential that those figures are sufficiently
thoughtful and benign: 'Individuals whose primary objects are
unloving and cruel may find the contemplation of the contents of
the mind of the object unbearable' (Fonagy 1991: 650). In consequence, the representation of mental events, of the child's own and
others' mental states, does not develop.

Fonagy then elaborates on the implications of this for understanding the abnormalities in mental processing which underlie
borderline personality disorder; without the capacity to conceive
the contents of one's own, as well as the object's mind, the
borderline child or adult may be protected from the intolerable
anxiety and pain of experiencing themselves as the object of hostile
intentions from those they love and depend on. The price is that
they are incapable of self-reflection and of attributing meaning to
their own feelings and other people's behaviour, which can only be
directly experienced and cannot be reflected upon or thought about
(Fonagy 1991; Fonagy *et al.* 1995).

Fonagy (1991) suggests that in borderline functioning, the failure of reflective function is self-imposed and partial, brought about by 'a defensive disavowal of the mental existence (in terms of psychic functioning) of the object'. Such disavowal is undertaken in the face of anticipation of unbearable psychic pain and consists of the obliteration of the significance of things while retaining their perception.

The 'significance of things' consists of the information which is stored in memory and which, when retrieved, provides a framework which organizes and gives meaning to a current event and current perceptions. When reflective function is deficient or absent it becomes impossible to link events into a meaningful narrative and intentionality, appraisal and separateness are also impossible.

Reflective function and its links with other theoretical concepts

The concept of reflective function is one which seems to encompass several key features which have been described in other theoretical frameworks. However, reflective function offers the most comprehensive explanation in that it is a description of a psychological capacity which can be demonstrated empirically and which can be traced back to its developmental roots in the emergence of theory of mind and even earlier to the pattern of interactions between mother and baby described by Gergely and Watson (1996).

Ego function

There are significant similarities between the concept of the ego and that of reflective function – both are descriptions of appraisal mechanisms for evaluating the significance of an experience. However, a crucial difference between them reflects a theme that emerges from time to time throughout this book, namely the move in analytic understanding from an account of mental structures to one of mental processes. The ego is described as a psychic structure, whereas reflective function is a more dynamic concept, in that it is a process which includes the constant evaluation of the pattern of relationship between self and other. Appraisal is an activity undertaken by the whole mind rather than by one part of it and the concept of reflective function therefore avoids the danger of identifying one part of the mind such as the ego as 'a homunculus', a mind within a mind (Cortina 2003).

Mirroring

Reflective function is a more subtle account of mirroring, a term used in somewhat different ways by psychoanalysts. Kohut describes the patient's need to be mirrored as 'to be looked upon with joy and basic approval by a delighted parental selfobject' (Kohut 1984: 143). This use of the term emphasizes the emotional response of the parent and, while most analysts agree that this is essential for healthy development, it does not capture the cognitive aspect of mirroring conveyed in the term reflective function, the fact that empathy is not just love and admiration but an active relating to the infant's mental processes and a constant attempt to see meaning in his or her communications.

Lacan's mirror stage is one of mutual identification, a merging of self and other (Lemaire 1977: 79), rather than a recognition of self and of one's separate subjectivity. Winnicott (1971) differentiates his ideas about mirroring from those of Lacan, in that he sees mirroring as an experience in which the infant gradually acquires a sense of subjectivity, with a central role given to the mother's face:

> What does the baby see when he or she looks at the mother's face? I am suggesting that, ordinarily, what the baby sees is himself or herself. In other words the mother is looking at the baby and *what she looks like is related to what she sees there*.
> (Winnicott 1971: 112, original emphasis)

He goes on to explore the impact on the baby who looks at the mother and does not see him- or herself because the mother is preoccupied and unresponsive for one reason or another and suggests that in these circumstances the baby's creative capacity begins to atrophy. There are many respects in which Winnicott's model of mirroring is the closest to the attachment theory concept of reflective function, especially in that he gives central importance to the mother's responsiveness to the baby's capacity to develop a sense of meaning and purpose, in other words the capacity for appraisal and intentionality which are key aspects of reflective function.

Alpha function

Reflective function has many features in common with Bion's (1962) concepts of maternal reverie and of the mother's alpha function, by which the infant's meaningless beta elements are transformed into alpha elements, which in turn become the building blocks of symbolic thought. An attuned mother intuitively puts her own psyche at the infant's disposal, as a container into which the infant can then project his bodily sensations. The mother endows these with subjective meaning so that the infant can take them back as psychological as well as physical experiences. A crucial feature of reflective function is that the mother attributes intentionality to her infant, thus enabling the infant gradually to find his own mind, to become aware of his own psychic processes and to form mental models of himself as a psychological and emotional being with wishes, desires, intentions and beliefs.

Transcendent function

Bovensiepen (2002) has noted the similarity between Jung's concept of the transcendent function and Bion's alpha function, and transcendent function can also be related to reflective function. Transcendent function describes the capacity to symbolize and so to find new meanings in experience and in the unconscious. In his essay on the transcendent function, Jung wrote:

> The present day shows with appalling clarity how little able people are to let the other man's argument count, although this capacity is a fundamental and indispensible condition for any human community. Everyone who proposes to come to terms with himself must reckon with this basic problem. For to the degree that he does not admit the validity of the other person, he denies the 'other' within himself the right to exist and vice-versa. The capacity for inner dialogue is a touchstone for outer objectivity.
>
> (Jung 1957[1916]: para. 187)

In this statement Jung describes the unconscious as the 'other', recognizing that it may be projected onto another person and related to in that person rather than in oneself. However, Jung was using the term 'transcendent function' to describe a person's ability to tolerate difference, an openness to alternative opinions and beliefs, not only in other people but also in oneself. Jung wrote: 'the shuttling to and fro of arguments represents the transcendent function of opposites' (Jung 1957[1916]: para. 189).

In attachment theory it is the development of this capacity which defines reflective function, in that reflective function depends upon the awareness that other people have minds of their own with beliefs and judgements that may differ from one's own and that cannot be dismissed or treated as insignificant. Both transcendent function and reflective function are descriptions of the capacity to relate to other people as psychologically as well as physically separate. The concept of transcendent function would therefore seem to resonate with the aspects of reflective function that relate to psychological separateness – or individuation which was Jung's own term for this process.

Feeling function

Jung recognized how important it is to be able to evaluate experiences and to make judgements about them. He described this as the 'feeling' function, which enables a person to decide on the value of an event or an experience. Appraisal is a key feature of reflective function and has been increasingly recognized by cognitive scientists as a constant unconscious process by which experiences are constantly screened and evaluated to determine their meaning and significance. Unfortunately Jung's pioneering work in identifying the importance of this process of appraisal goes largely unrecognized by those who now investigate the process from information-processing and neurophysiological perspectives. This may partly arise from the frequent misuse of the term 'feeling function' by analytical psychologists themselves. Ann Casement (2001) points out that 'in particular all kinds of fictions congregate around the *feeling* function. The latter, along with the *thinking* function, is a way of evaluating so that something is seen as being "good" or "bad", "nice" or "nasty", "beautiful" or "ugly"' (Casement 2001: 132, original emphasis). She suggests that many different connotations of the word 'feeling' in the English language contribute to the misunderstanding of Jung's use of the word to mean appraisal or evaluation.

Conclusions

I have explored in this chapter the relationship between the concept
of reflective function and several other theoretical models in psychoanalysis and analytical psychology. I have suggested that
reflective function offers a higher order theory which encompasses
the key features of all the other models which attempt to explain
how the human mind evaluates and finds meaning in experience.
Reflective function describes a dynamic process which is not
limited to a structural or topographical part of the mind in contrast
to the concept of ego. Reflective function is an activity undertaken
by the whole mind, conscious and unconscious, rather than by one
part of it.

The developmental roots of reflective function can be demonstrated by the experiments which show the increasingly complex
and sophisticated awareness of theory of mind in children as they
grow up. The concepts of alpha function, mirroring and transcendent function do not have their roots in such a clearly defined
developmental pathway. The benefits of parents' reflective function
and the psychological difficulties experienced by children of parents
who show insufficient reflective function have also been demonstrated empirically.

However, there is another dimension to this discussion of reflective function, a dimension which partly reflects and partly acts as
counter to much of what I have written so far in this chapter. It
seems clear that there are times when reflective function becomes
too painful for the human mind to tolerate. The developmental
achievement of theory of mind and of reflective function requires an
awareness of mental separateness, that we are each truly alone in
the world, and this can feel like a mental and emotional isolation
which is intolerable and which can only partly be overcome by
means of empathy and projection. Reflective function is like the
apple from the tree of knowledge in the garden of Eden – once it has
been eaten, it becomes impossible to return to infantile paradise
where there is no self-knowledge, no awareness of separateness.

I think that this is a form of loneliness which may contribute to
the fascination that stories of doomed romantic love hold for so
many of us, because these stories contain two key features. First,
they usually convey a sense of two people gripped by a powerful
force over which they have no control and which leaves them no
choice but to submit to its power. The relationship is experienced as

destiny or fate and neither of the fated pair can resist it. Romeo's sense of fate is conveyed in his remark: 'Some consequence yet hanging in the stars shall bitterly begin his fearful date with this night's revels and expire the term of a despised life closed in my breast by some vile forfeit of untimely death' (Shakespeare, *Romeo and Juliet*, Act 1, Scene 4).

The second point is that, as Romeo seems to know, the passionate relationship inevitably leads to death for the two lovers; to fall out of love or to become an ordinary couple, growing old together, each relating to the other as a separate and independent person seems impossible for the lovers to contemplate. Juliet says to Romeo as he climbs down from her balcony: 'Methinks I see thee now thou art so low as one dead in the bottom of a tomb' (*Romeo and Juliet*, Act 3, Scene 5). The relationship is one of fusion, and fusion requires the destruction of an independent identity and so of reflective function, eventually leading to the complete mindlessness of death.

The fatalistic love stories of Romeo and Juliet, Lancelot and Guinevere, Tristan and Isolde may express our longing at times to revert to a kind of mindlessness, in which an intensity of emotion carries one along without thought, self-awareness or reflection. However, these love stories also spell out the price that has to be paid for the passionate fusion with another, in which the sense of oneself as a separate being is lost. The price is the abandonment of reflective function, an abandonment that obliterates the mind as an internal object, and this is psychological death.

Chapter 7

The process of change in analysis and the role of the analyst

The developmental approach to the human psyche, which has been the main theme and focus of this book so far, can also help us to investigate the analytic process itself. Just as representation, symbolism and meaning are emergent features of the astonishingly complex interaction of the genome, the brain and the interpersonal world of the human infant, so intrapsychic change during analytic therapy, with the creation of new symbols and meanings, can also be seen to emerge out of the complex interactions between the conscious and unconscious of both analyst and analysand.

The discussion which follows will highlight some of the issues which have recurred throughout the book so far, such as the relative role of actual experience or of autonomous unconscious mechanisms in contributing to intrapsychic change. The analyst's interpretations, for example, are real events which, in the structural model in psychoanalysis, are internalized and gradually modify the psychic structures of the ego, superego and id. In analytical psychology, on the other hand, the classical approach has been that the analytic process serves to activate innate archetypal imagery which instigates a self-healing process in the psyche, with the external world playing a relatively minor role.

The central issue at stake here is that our understanding of the ways in which the mind works underpins our views of the ways in which analysis brings about psychic change in our patients. Psychodynamic theories can be accurate only if their elements correspond to the actual cognitive capacities of the human, both in infancy and in adulthood, and also if they accurately reflect the developmental processes out of which the complexity of the human psyche and its representations arise. Does the concept of the archetype as an image schema, for example, have any impact on the way we practise clinically? Does it change the nature of our interpretations if we think that the unconscious consists of internal working models rather than drive-based internal objects and that repression provides only one explanation for the inaccessibility of some information to conscious awareness? One of the most important developments in the last 20 years has been the convergence of research findings from across a spectrum of related disciplines, including developmental psychology, neurobiology and attachment theories, showing that the cognitive and emotional development of the human mind is not solipsistic but crucially depends on interpersonal relationships, from the earliest weeks of life onwards and even *in utero* (Schore 1994; Stern 1985; Piontelli 1992). It is this approach which has been predominant in this book so far and which informs the study of the process of analytic change in this chapter.

Many analysts, both psychoanalysts and analytical psychologists, argue that compatibility with the research from other disciplines is unimportant for analytic theories. Such an analyst will continue to use a theoretical model if it continues to provide meaningful and useful explanations for the analyst and, through the analyst's interpretations, for the patient. If such a consistent model is also accompanied by therapeutic improvement, the analyst may continue to use the model without needing to investigate its compatibility with the cognitive capacities and developmental mechanisms demonstrated by empirical research. Within each school of analytic thought there are some analysts who remain resolute in their beliefs that their model of the psyche is the true one.

The problem of analytic diversity: too many narratives

In spite of the impression conveyed by some analysts that there is only one true model for the process of analytic change, the range of views across the analytic spectrum shows that, in reality, a century of theory and practice in both psychoanalysis and analytical psychology have produced great variety and disparity. Freudian, Jungian, Kleinian and attachment theorists all envisage the goals of analytic therapy differently in terms of the changes which may be brought about in the psyche. Sandler and Dreher (1996) emphasize this point:

Consider for a moment, the frequently stated formulation that the aim of analysis is to bring about structural change. Yet the meaning of such a statement will be dependent on whether it is looked at from the point of view of, for instance, ego psychology, self psychology or object-relations theory; moreover we would have to ask which structure is involved. Is change being considered in relation to superego, ego, mental representations or relations to internal objects?

(Sandler and Dreher 1996: 114)

They have given a detailed historical account of the changes that have taken place within Freudian theory and practice in terms of the goals for change in psychoanalysis and have concluded that 'a desirable outcome of analysis will vary from one patient to another, and is not capable of being encompassed by one definition or measured by one single criterion' (Sandler and Dreher 1996: 122).

However, there is a problem with this pluralistic approach in which there are many stories, any of which may be true at a particular moment, a problem which has been highlighted by Arlow (1996), who argues that the theoretical standpoint of an analyst determines his interpretation of the patient's material:

each will orient himself differently to the patient's productions, selectively attending and responding to those elements that are consonant with his theory of pathogenesis. Each will find a different psychic reality in keeping with the favoured view of what processes or events they believe caused neurotic illness and character deformation. Under the circumstances, therefore the concept of psychic reality furnishes no common ground for discourse. It has become an anachronism.

(Arlow 1996: 664)

This has been graphically illustrated by a study in which the researchers tried to assess the degree to which an analytic process (AP) could be said to be occurring in analytic sessions (Vaughan *et al.* 1997). The Columbia Analytic Process Scale (CAPS) was used to assess the extent to which free association, interpretation and working through took place in analytic sessions; although the CAPS had good inter-rater reliability, it was not possible to establish its construct validity because among the senior training analysts involved in the project, no clinical consensus as to the presence of AP could be established. Analysts agreed that it was a vital part of the analytic process, but there was 'no meaningful consensual definition of the term AP among a group of training and supervising analysts from the Columbia Center for Psychoanalytic Training and Research' (Vaughan *et al.* 1997: 964). It is likely that the criteria which analysts use to identify AP are still too primitive to give an accurate or clear account of that process.

If it is not even possible to agree on what constitutes the fundamental process in analytic therapy there can be no hope of demonstrating that any therapeutic gain may result from that process rather than from other non-specific factors, such as the intensity of sessions; there is also no hope of investigating the relative merits of different theoretical models in bringing about the analytic process, if analysts cannot even agree on whether AP is taking place. It therefore may not be possible to make a judgement about the validity of one model of psychic reality over another on clinical grounds, in that all models may be clinically useful and appear to account for psychic change at different times. Soren Ekstrom (2002) has adopted a constructive approach to this analytic diversity, suggesting that 'the only meaningful way to describe therapy interactions is as two-way communication: as patient narratives, analyst narratives and, more tentatively, as therapeutic narratives' (Ekstrom 2002: 354). He argues that therapists should embrace the fact that our understanding of our patients' lives is story based and that we need to use our own stories when we listen to and respond to our patients' narratives.

Developments in psychoanalytic theory and technique

Some psychoanalysts strongly resist what they consider to be a dangerous encroachment of knowledge from other fields of inquiry. André Green, for example, has written:

> Observation cannot tell us anything about intrapsychic processes that truly characterize the subject's experience [and that the analytic setting] provides an opportunity to observe and participate in a unique form of mental functioning, which is the only way through which the analytic state of mind can be

experienced, integrated and tested, year after year, day after day, hour after hour.

(Green 2001: 71–2)

Donald Meltzer (1973) adopts a similar position in relation to transference interpretation:

> On the basis of validated hypotheses about the here-and-now transference and using his inference from the compulsion to repeat, the analyst may construct the development of the unconscious object relations of the patient. From a wide experience of individual patients he may then generalize and propose a theory of development which he believes to be biologically founded on the deep levels of the psyche and not fundamentally different in varying races, or circumstances of life.

(Meltzer 1973: 12)

These analysts seem to assume that the psychoanalytic method of investigation can itself produce an accurate scientific model of the human mind and that information from more objective sources of investigation is superfluous; they would argue that the psycho-analytic method provides the only access to unconscious contents, but fail to see that their own preconceptions determine the way in which such unconscious material is interpreted. They do not appreciate that the clinical material which they understand in terms of one theoretical model might be interpreted in terms of a completely different conceptual framework.

The increasing evidence available from other disciplines about the ways in which the mind encodes, categorizes, stores and retrieves information cannot be so easily dismissed. It leads to an increasing questioning of the belief that is central to Freud's model, that there is only one proper analytic technique, that of inter-preting repressed unconscious material and the accompanying defences. For many psychoanalysts, anything else has been con-sidered to be, at worst, suggestion, and at best a deviation from correct technique. There are a number of psychoanalysts who still adopt this approach. Hannah Segal (1986[1981]: 10), for example, writes: 'A full interpretation of an unconscious phantasy involves all its aspects. It has to be traced to its original instinctual source, so that the impulses underlying the phantasy are laid bare'. She continues: 'These deeper layers must be taken into consideration if we are to understand the analysand's anxieties and the structure of his internal world, the basis of which is laid in early infancy' (Segal 1986[1981]: 10). Another psychoanalyst strongly argues that 'only analytical interpretation can lead to the patient's correct insight into the unconscious pathogens of his psychoneurosis' (Kerz-Rühling 1996: 228).

Some of the roots of the attitude I have just described lie in the history of the psychoanalytic movement. Hamilton (1996) points out that the close connection between hypnosis and transference led Freud and his colleagues strenuously to avoid any possible accusation that suggestion might be a causal factor in bringing about change in analysis. Hamilton writes:

> Since Freud, psychoanalysts have made concerted efforts to purify the field and their professional lives of this unwelcome 'contaminant'. Ultimately these efforts have meant that some psychoanalytic practitioners have attempted to rid the psychoanalytic encounter of its relational – that is, emotional or affective – properties.
>
> (Hamilton 1996: 23)

Hamilton concludes that this attempt to 'study humans as if they were not human beings but, rather, mental structures, underlying principles, biological forces or affective outbursts' has led psychoanalysts to introduce a whole set of 'extra "non-analytic" ideas, such as the "real relationship", the holding environment, "parameters", supportive techniques, to account for what most of them find themselves doing and saying, their theories notwithstanding' (Hamilton 1996: 23). These techniques are seen as necessary deviations from the pure analytic method and by defining them as extra-analytic, the core concepts of analytic technique are somehow preserved.

There have been major divergences from this view in the newer psychoanalytic models such as self-psychology and the relational school of psychoanalysis. Both of these place the relationship with the analyst at the heart of the analytic experience and consider that it plays a vital part in bringing about intrapsychic change, although there are significant differences between these two models. Kohut's (1984) self-psychology still places interpretation at the heart of the process of analytic change, even though he offers a very different kind of interpretation from that of classical psychoanalysis. Kohut criticizes classical psychoanalytic technique as moralistic in its focus on the interpretation of instinctual drives, suggesting that this approach may repeat the essential trauma of childhood in a way that is harmful to the progress of the analysis. He suggests instead that it is vital for the analyst 'to acknowledge the validity and legitimacy of the patient's demands for development enhancing self–object responses'. An analyst who works in this way

> sets in motion a process which, via the optimal frustrations to which the analyst exposes the patient through more or less accurate and timely interpretations, leads to the transmuting internalization of the self-object analyst and his functions and thus to the acquisition of psychic structure.
>
> (Kohut 1984: 172)

While the relational aspects are therefore acknowledged as crucial in self-psychology, Kohut argues that interpretation is still the central tool at the analyst's disposal.

In contrast, the relational school tends, on the whole, to view the analytic experience as sometimes mutative in itself. Interpretation is not the gold standard of analytic technique, indeed it may even be counter-productive at times, according to the late Stephen Mitchell, one of whose last publications was his response to a *Journal of Analytical Psychology* questionnaire designed and edited by the journal's US editor, Joe Cambray. Mitchell emphasized the fact that

> there is no way for the analyst not to act, and, in one way or another, to re-enact as well. What is crucial is a continual self-reflection on the dense, multiple reverberations of the past in the present and a commitment to forms of interaction that seem most enhancing to the patient's developing vitality and sense of freedom.
>
> (Mitchell 2002: 87)

He goes on to suggest that sometimes interpretations may generate self-consciousness in the less desirable sense of awkwardness and self-preoccupation and that part of what was healing about a particular patient's experiences with him was 'precisely that they had an erotic dimension to them, a shared pleasure that was accepted between us and unremarked upon' (Mitchell 2002: 87). Ted Jacobs and James Fosshage both share this view in their responses to the same questionnaire. James Fosshage (2002) high-lights the crucial importance of a balance between interpretation and the exploration of new experience writing that 'the consistent emphasis on interpretation in psychoanalysis has tended to obfus-cate the importance of new relational experience' and argues that 'an analysis that is too exclusive in its use of exploration and interpretation will tend to limit the requisite co-creation of new experience' (Fosshage 2002: 76). Ted Jacobs (2002) adopts a similar position, suggesting that

> insight in a vacuum, in other words, is of limited value. Insight must be combined with an experience that allows the patient not only to recognize his automatic protective patterns but also to relinquish them because he gradually discovers through his relationship with his analyst that he no longer needs these defences.
>
> (Jacobs 2002: 18)

Sandler and Dreher (1996) have explored the increasing diversity of aims formulated by the varying psychoanalytic schools and note that, paradoxically, the greater variety of theoretical formulations of aims has been accompanied by a degree of underlying similarity of the different approaches clinically. Weinshel (1990) argued that one of the areas of agreement has been a gradual movement towards a more modest conceptualization of psychoanalysis, whose aims have become increasingly realistic and more in harmony with clinical observations. Sandler and Dreher (1996) illustrate this with a summary of the range of the goals of contemporary psycho-analysis.

Psychoanalytic 'cures' are rarely spoken of. Psychic conflict cannot be completely eliminated,

> nor is the idea maintained that a 'complete' analysis is possible. Transferences cannot be completely eliminated or resolved. While insight is aimed for, it is no longer regarded as an absolutely necessary requirement, without which the analysis cannot proceed. The retrieval of repressed childhood memories

is no longer the main aim of the analytic work. On the other hand, over the years, analysis is now regarded as aiming to bring about intrapsychic changes which would result in improved resolution of the patient's main conflicts. While analyses are never complete, and transference can never be completely resolved, the analysis can still be seen as successful. Instead of aiming at insight, attainment of the capacity for self-observation is to be aimed for.

(Sandler and Dreher 1996: 114–15)

Jungian perspectives on the process of change in analysis

Jung (1939) referred to two processes of psychic change, one of which he called 'integration' and the other 'individuation'. Integration is essentially the process of making unconscious contents conscious and, on the whole, Jung seemed willing to accept a Freudian account of this process, although he emphasized the fact that repression is not the only mechanism by which psychic contents are kept out of consciousness:

Modern psychologists, too, tend to regard the unconscious as an ego-less function below the threshold of consciousness. Unlike the philosophers, they tend to derive its subliminal functions from the conscious mind. Janet thinks that there is a certain weakness of consciousness which is unable to hold all the psychic processes together. Freud on the other hand, favours the idea of conscious factors that suppress certain incompatible tendencies. Much can be said for both theories, since there are numerous cases where a weakness of consciousness actually causes certain contents to fall below the threshold or where disagreeable contents are repressed . . . Neurotic contents can be integrated without appreciable injury to the ego, but psychotic contents cannot.

(Jung 1939: para. 492)

With these statements, Jung seems to accept both dissociation and repression as mechanisms which can keep psychic material out of conscious awareness and his concept of integration could therefore be considered to refer to processes which overcome dissociation and those which overcome repression and so to be similar to psychoanalytic theory in this respect.

In contrast to some of the enduring strands in psychoanalytic theory which I have highlighted above, Jungian theory has recognized the relational aspects of therapy from the start. Jung was adamant that an effective analysis required the analyst to be affected and altered as well as the patient. He wrote:

> For since the analytical work must inevitably lead sooner or later to a fundamental discussion between 'I' and 'You' and 'You' and 'I' on a plane stripped of all human pretences, it is very likely, indeed it is almost certain, that not only the patient but the doctor as well will find the situation 'getting under his skin'. Nobody can meddle with fire or poison without being affected in some vulnerable spot; for the true physician does not stand outside his work but is always in the thick of it.
>
> (Jung 1944: para. 5)

As Christopher Perry (1997) points out in his study of Jungian perspectives on transference and countertransference, Jung fully recognized the importance of the transference and, in contrast to Freud, he also realized that the countertransference is a vital therapeutic tool in analysis. Perry writes that:

> whilst being alert to the potentially deleterious effects of countertransference, Jung also characteristically opened himself to the gradual realization that countertransference is a 'highly important organ of information' for the analyst.
>
> (Perry 1997: 142)

Jung's view was that analysis is a dialectical process 'in which the doctor, as a person, participates just as much as the patient' (Jung 1951: para. 239). This was the basis of Jung's view that analysts must first have had a thorough training analysis themselves, although he was under no illusion that this would be 'an absolutely certain means of dispelling illusions and projections', but he argued that it would at least develop the capacity for self-criticism. He went on to suggest that 'a good half of every treatment that probes at all deeply consists in the doctor's examining of himself, for only what

he can put right in himself can he hope to put right in the patient'
and proposed this as the true meaning of the concept of the
'wounded physician' (Jung 1951: para. 239). This view culminated
in his diagram of the counter-crossing conscious and unconscious transference and countertransference relationships that he
explored in alchemical terms and that emerge in analysis (Jung
1946: para. 422).

However, there are some other aspects of Jung's model which, at
first sight, appear to conflict with the interpersonal view of the
analytic process. Another key feature of Jung's model for the
process of change in analysis is the active, creative and constructive
role that he attributed to the unconscious in analysis. Jung's view
was that the sources of the creative power of the unconscious were
the collective unconscious and the archetypes, especially the
archetype of the self which is a unifying and integrating principle
within the psyche. I have discussed the various ways in which Jung
thought about archetypes in Chapter 2 and his concept of the self
shares in this confusion to some extent, in that he sometimes
describes the self as the centre of personality, sometimes as the
total of all aspects of the psyche and sometimes as an archetype.
Fordham (1963) has explored the theoretical incompatibilities in
Jung's writings about the self and has proposed that the 'self'
should be considered as the totality of the psyche and has suggested that, in addition, there is a central archetype of order, which
organizes the unconscious (Fordham 1963).

Jung emphatically rejected the idea that analysis should consist
solely of a one-way relationship between conscious and unconscious parts of the mind. The concept of 'individuation' is the term
Jung coined to describe a separate process for bringing about
psychological change and he argued that it is in this process that
the unconscious plays an active and creative role. Jung was quite
specific that the purpose of analysis is to allow a person's sense of
identity to enlarge to encompass unconscious material, a process
which he named individuation and defined as:

> the process by which a person becomes a psychological 'in-
> dividual', that is, a separate, indivisible unity or 'whole'. It is
> generally assumed that consciousness is the whole of the
> psychological individual. But knowledge of the phenomena
> that can only be explained on the hypothesis of unconscious

psychic processes makes it doubtful whether the ego and its contents are in fact identical with the 'whole'.

(Jung 1939: para. 490)

He made clear that the concept of 'whole' must necessarily include not only consciousness but the illimitable field of unconscious occurrences as well and later, in the same section, wrote:

Conscious and unconscious do not make a whole when one of them is suppressed and injured by the other. If they must contend, let it at least be a fair fight with equal rights on both sides. Both are aspects of life. Consciousness should defend its reason and protect itself and the chaotic life of the unconscious should be given the chance of having its way too – as much of it as we can stand . . . This, roughly, is what I mean by the individuation process. As the name shows it is a process or course of development arising out of the conflict between the two fundamental psychic facts . . .

How the harmonising of conscious and unconscious data is to be undertaken cannot be indicated in the form of a recipe . . . Out of this union emerge new situations and new conscious attitudes. I have therefore called the union of opposites 'the transcendent function'. This rounding out of the personality into a whole may well be the goal of any psychotherapy that claims to be more than a mere cure of symptoms.

(Jung 1939: paras 522–4)

With statements such as this, Jung supported his view of the psyche as self-regulating, with neurotic symptoms and dreams operating as communications from the unconscious, to compensate for an unbalanced conscious attitude. Anthony Storr (1983) has pointed out that this concept runs through the whole of Jung's scheme of how the mind works, underpinning his classification of psychological types and has summarized this with great clarity:

In Western man, because of the achievements of his culture, there was an especial tendency towards intellectual hubris; an overvaluation of thinking which could alienate a man from his emotional roots. Neurotic symptoms, dreams and other manifestations of the unconscious were often expressions of the 'other side' trying to assert itself. There was, therefore, within every individual, a striving towards unity in which divisions would be replaced by consistency, opposites equally balanced, consciousness in reciprocal relation with the unconscious.

(Storr 1983: 18)

This concept of self-regulation therefore lies at the heart of the individuation process and of the process of change in analysis, which can help to bring about a new synthesis between conscious and unconscious. Jung wrote:

> If the unconscious can be recognized as a co-determining factor along with consciousness, and if we can live in such a way that conscious and unconscious demands are taken into account as far as possible, then the centre of gravity of the total personality shifts its position. It is no longer in the ego, which is merely the centre of consciousness, but in the hypothetical point between conscious and unconscious. This new centre might be called the self.
>
> (Jung 1967: para. 67)

Storr offers a way of reconciling this apparent contradiction between the impact of interpersonal experience and autonomous intrapsychic processes in Jung's model of psychic change:

> In times when so much importance is attributed to good or bad interpersonal relationships as determinants of mental health or illness, Jung's concentration upon the individual's relations with the different parts of his own psyche may seem puzzling. Jung was well aware of the importance of interpersonal relationships, but believed that it was only when the individual had come to terms with himself that satisfactory relationships with others could be achieved.
>
> (Storr 1983: 22)

Contemporary Jungians have subsequently developed Jung's models for the process of change in analytic therapy to include childhood experience, offering, in the developmental model that largely originated in the work of Michael Fordham, a more complete reconciliation of the apparent contradiction between the role of the archetype and that of interpersonal experience. Fordham revolutionized analytical psychology with his reformulation of the concept of the self to include the idea of an original self which deintegrates, to originate development in infancy, initiating a cycle of deintegration and reintegration:

> [I]n essence deintegration and reintegration describe a fluctu-
> ating state of learning in which the infant opens itself to new
> experiences and then withdraws in order to reintegrate and
> consolidate those experiences. During a deintegrative activity,
> the infant maintains continuity with the main body of the self
> (or its centre) while venturing into the external world to accu-
> mulate experience in motor action and sensory stimulation.
>
> (Fordham 1988: 64)

The work of Piontelli (1992) suggests that this is a process that probably begins even before birth, a view accepted by contemporary analytical psychologists. Gordon (1993) has clarified the developmental relationship between archetypal imagery and personal experience:

> in the course of development the archetypal figures become
> tamed by being incarnated in and through actual relationships
> to actual persons; these persons come gradually to be perceived
> with more or less accuracy in terms of their actual nature
> and character. In other words, they become more humanized.
> Perceptions become more appropriate, less ruthless, more
> compassionate; the archetypal projections are withdrawn, and
> the capacity for truth emerges. And then both the paradisal
> and the terrifying worlds begin to recede.
>
> (Gordon 1993: 303)

Another key paper that represents this developmental approach was entitled 'The indivisibility of the personal and the collective unconscious' (Williams 1963). Williams suggests that 'nothing in the personal unconscious needs to be repressed unless the ego feels threatened by its archetypal power' and that the archetypal activity which forms the individual's myth is dependent on material supplied by the personal unconscious (Williams 1963: 79). The developmental model that underpins this view is also one that accurately describes the process of change in analysis, as Fordham himself clearly stated, writing that 'one manifestation of deinteg-ration is the making of interpretation with conviction' (Fordham 1985: 126).

An attachment theory perspective on the process of change in analysis

An attachment theory perspective has far-reaching implications for our models of the process of change in analysis, for analytical psychologists as well as for psychoanalysts, and I shall now move on to investigate some of these. An attachment theory paradigm may be able to resolve the dilemma about the relative importance of the interpretative and the relational perspectives of analytic practice, providing a coherent information-processing framework in which both have equal weight and validity.

In essence, it is the concepts of implicit memory and the internal working model which provide the basis for a paradigm shift in relation to our understanding of the human psyche; if information is inaccessible to consciousness, not because it is actively repressed but simply because it is encoded and stored in a format that is unavailable to consciousness, then the idea that such material can be made conscious by the analyst's interpretation which overcomes repression, is doomed to failure.

An attachment theory/information processing account of change in analysis includes three key features.

- *State-dependent retrieval:* the analytic experience activates internal working models of past relationships with key attach-ment figures (see pp. 82–4). These are actively relived in the present relationship with the analyst, usually without awareness that the present experience is being distorted by the powerful patterns of expectations and emotions which form a key part of the activated implicit memories.
- *The development of narrative competence:* the overcoming of dissociative defences and the integration of dissociated internal working models. Implicit memories are activated and experi-enced in the here-and-now, in the transference and integrated with episodic memories of past experience and relationships.
- *Formation of new internal working models:* these form the basis for a move from insecure to secure attachments, and an increase in reflective function.

State-dependent retrieval

In the analytic situation, patients reveal considerable personal information, often of an emotionally painful nature and often reflecting negative self-perceptions; this disclosure, together with the lack of objective information about their analyst's personality, attitudes and interests, leads patients to draw on internal working models of their childhood patterns of relationship to parents in order to give meaning to their perceptions of their analyst. Thus, patients whose pattern of attachments was insecure in childhood will bring the same pattern of insecure attachments to the analytic relationship and will start to relate to their analyst in the same way as they did to their parents. This may also form the necessary emotional state which brings about state-dependent retrieval of specific autobiographical memories, with accompanying emotions. These are explicit or episodic memories which are actively relived in the analysis as the underlying internal working models are retrieved. The 'explicit' memories may also provide useful historical evidence for analysts which can enable them to identify more accurately the pattern of interpersonal relationship with their patients which they experience in the analysis. Conway (1990) has conducted experiments which demonstrate that 'emotion concepts are represented in memory by exemplars and the exemplars are primarily autobiographical memories of emotional experiences' (Conway 1990: 142). Conway's experiments involved verbal reporting and could demonstrate only what is stored in 'explicit' or 'declarative' memory; they did not investigate the role of implicit memory in storing information about past emotional experience.

However, Fonagy (1999a) has argued that it is not the retrieval of these historical explicit memories which brings about change in analysis, but rather that '[t]herapeutic work needs to focus on helping the patient identify regular patterns of behaviour and fantasy based on childhood fantasy and experience, for which autobiographical memory can provide no explanation' (Fonagy 1999a: 220). He argues that implicit memory stores patterns of relating as psychic structures organizing behaviour saying that 'it is these structures and not the events that give rise to them that need to be the focus of psychoanalytic work' (Fonagy 1999a: 220). Fonagy's ideas suggest that explicit autobiographical memories are illustrative of past experiences but that the retrieval of, and conscious attention to, these explicit memories do not in themselves bring about change; instead it is the retrieval of internal working models which provides the essential foundation stone for intra-psychic change.

This is, of course, very familiar to all analysts and psycho-therapists through their work with the transference, the uncon-scious attitudes and expectations that the patient holds towards the analyst and which result from the projections of internal attachment figures and patterns of relationship from that person's past life. Projection in general can be envisaged as the activation of internal working models, usually of childhood patterns of rela-tionship with parents as I described in Chapter 4. Once retrieved, these internal working models of past experiences, then organize and structure that person's experience in the present and so form the basis for a range of distorted perceptions of the analyst which may be vividly lived through and enacted in the transference.

Furthermore, the internal working models underpin subtle patterns of behaviour which can exert a powerful 'pull' in the recipient of these projections, in this case the analyst, who may feel under considerable pressure to enact the part attributed to him or her, an experience which is usually described as projective identi-fication. The patient's unconscious expectations and the accom-panying unconscious signals can seem to act as a kind of script which it can be very difficult for the analyst to recognize and resist. Eagle (1995) suggests that this identification of the pressures on the analyst is one of the central parts of analytic work:

> Among the most important functions of the therapist in the treatment situation are (1) the need to be aware of the responses 'pulled for' from him or her; (2) the importance of not responding to the patient in accord with these demands; and (3) bringing these demands to the patient's awareness and examining the sequence of event and interactions that has occurred.
>
> (Eagle 1995: 138)

However, there is another aspect to state-dependent retrieval that analysts may be more reluctant to acknowledge, namely the possi-bility that there may be some very real aspects to their own behaviour or attitudes that the patient accurately detects and which therefore mean that the patient's projection is not a distortion but a psychic mechanism which accurately identifies real features of the therapist's personality. Therapists need to have a high degree of both self-awareness and humility to recognize the times when the patient's perception of them is accurate and, at times, to confirm this to the patient. A relational model makes it much easier and less persecutory for analysts to accept and admit this when it happens, but therapists may also have to face the fact that they may have reached the limits of their abilities or may need further analysis or supervision themselves.

The development of narrative competence

Integration of dissociated working models

In Chapter 5, I explored an attachment theory model of psychic defences, suggesting that persistent avoidance of the painful meanings of memories or experiences is initially based on a process of conscious suppression which then becomes automatic, in the form of repression and finally leads to dissociation, in which different clusters of memories, attitudes, emotions and self-representations become dissociated from each other in separate and unintegrated internal working models. This is thought to be one of the key features of borderline personality disorder, in which marked changes in mood, attitude and personality reflect the underlying switch from the predominance of one set of internal working models to another. In its most extreme form, multiple personality disorder is a condition in which the personality change seems to be total, as though there really are several different people contained in one body. I need to point out here that this is one of the two forms of dissociation which I outlined in Chapter 5; the other is the immediate dissociation brought about by trauma, in which information is encoded subcortically without conscious awareness, leading to the phenomena, such as flashbacks and amnesia, which reflect the automatic, state-dependent nature of these dissociated memories.

In analysis, part of the skill and art of being a therapist is the intuitive modulation of affect to a level which makes it possible for the patient to tolerate living through the painful emotions and attitudes to self and other that accompany the activation of a previously dissociated internal working model. As the analysand slowly discovers that it is possible to survive the disorientating experience of switching from one state to another, the analyst's role as modulator is gradually internalized and becomes part of a higher order internal working model which integrates fragmented self and object relations and the previously dissociated internal working models.

Integration of implicit memories with episodic memories

Each time that an autobiographical memory is talked about in an analytic session, the explicit memory is retrieved and becomes the focus for conscious attention. It may be an accurate memory of the original event which is retrieved, or it may be memories which contain a considerable amount of reconstruction of the event, if the patient has already spent quite a lot of time thinking about it and reworking the events in imagination, as I have described in Chapter 5. In analysis, recalling a particular memory is usually used as part of a process of finding meaningful patterns in past experience. I would suggest that the frequent rehearsal of autobiographical memories in analysis does play a key part in bringing about change in analysis, but not in the way that Freud initially envisaged, through the overcoming of repression. Instead I would suggest that the recollection and frequent description in analysis of an increasing number of autobiographical memories allow them to be compared and integrated with each other into a meaningful narrative. They can also act as signposts to the underlying internal working models and so provide a vehicle for the gradual integration of specific memories with the implicit patterns of past relationships.

CLINICAL ILLUSTRATION

A patient, an academic, is unable to produce written work, even though her career is severely adversely affected by this failure; her history strongly indicates that implicit memories of childhood relationships with critical parents or other authority figures play a major part in creating this writing block.

This patient's childhood experience was of a mother who was very ambitious for her daughter and expected very high achievements from her. All through her childhood, her parents had expected, not just high standards, but that she should be the best at school and so she was, coming in the top three in her year through the whole of her school career. Her mother was full of praise for my patient when she was successful at school, but became extremely punitive when she occasionally misbehaved at home. My patient remembers that she and her sister were made to kneel on the floor which had been scattered with small beans, which were very painful to kneel on; other painful punishments were imposed, often for some minor failing. At these times she felt terrified and helpless because she simply did not understand why her mother was being so cruel to her.

A more acute trauma occurred when she was aged about 4 and was changed from a class with a teacher she liked to a more advanced class where the teacher was clearly overtly sadistic; my patient was younger than the others and a little slower in copying letters and words off the blackboard. The teacher would rub the words out before she had finished and would then berate her in front of the whole class when she was unable to reproduce the words on the blackboard. My patient became terrified to go to school, but her mother would insist that she went and seemed unaware of the very real terror that she felt, until one day she was so frightened that she urinated on the floor in front of the whole class. She was in such distress that her mother finally recognized the severity of the situation and removed her.

This patient is doing research in a science field as a senior member of a research team, but she is on short-term funding and therefore effectively is totally dependent professionally on the professor who heads the research team. She now has to write two papers, accounts of experiments which have been completed, the data analysed and the only task left is the writing up, which she is unable to do. The longer she leaves it the worse the problem becomes, so that initially she cannot look at the work, then she cannot go into the office with the computer on which the work is stored, then she cannot go into the office at all and finally she cannot even get out of bed. She knows that eventually at the very last minute, when it is almost too late and when everyone is furious with her, she will finally force herself to sit down and write the papers: this is what has happened on several occasions before. It is important to note that all the work required for the paper has been completed and the problem is a very clearly defined one of writing it up.

In her young adult life, this patient had had no significant psychological problems until the time when she wrote her first research paper; her supervisor (who was newly appointed himself) severely criticized it in a harsh way which she found painful and humiliating. She lost a considerable amount of confidence at that point and from then onwards she began to have increasing difficulty in producing written work and would become depressed and lethargic, avoiding going to work altogether at times.

Her present phobic avoidance of writing would seem to have very clear origins in this experience, in her parents' over-high expectations of her, her own defences of omnipotent and grandiose feelings that she can perform better than everyone else and her terror of humiliation and punishment if she fails. The act of writing seems to create state-dependent retrieval, where the physical task of writing, in relation particularly to academic work which must be produced for critical appraisal, retrieves the memories of hostile authority figures who want to punish and humiliate her; it also retrieves the memories of her own mental distress which she experienced as a child of 4 and also when she produced her first research paper.

Her writing block occurs in a context where she feels belittled by her professor and she feels angry with and humiliated by him, so that these feelings also directly match those of past distressing mental processes. She has directly confirmed this by telling me at the start of the latest session that she noticed that the tightness she feels in her chest, and the sense of panic when she tries to sit at the computer and write, are exactly the same as the sensations she used to feel when she went to school terrified at age 4. It is important to note that my patient had not forgotten the childhood trauma which I have recounted above but avoided thinking about it, describing it to me and linking it with her present symptoms of panic and tightness in the chest, with considerable reluctance, only after she had been in therapy for many months.

The only way she can avoid this state-dependent retrieval of her own and other people's mental processes is not to write and in this way she succeeds in avoiding the state-dependent retrieval of memories which it is intolerable for her to contemplate because they contain information about sadistic and punitive mental processes in her primary school teacher and her first academic supervisor and also about her mother's lack of an empathic response to her distress.

During the therapy she has identified that her depression, emotional withdrawal and difficulty in writing are often triggered by criticism or by the fear of hostility from senior colleagues towards her or her work. She has become aware that she falls into a state of mind in which the world seems to be a dangerous and hostile place and that at any moment she may be attacked. It took her some months to recognize that this fear was the major factor causing her to feel so anxious and depressed and several more months to begin to link this pattern of present expectation with her past experience of an unpredictably cruel and hostile mother. It was not the specific autobiographical memories about her mother's behaviour which were structuring her present experience and leading her to expect similar hostility and cruelty from those in authority over her, but unconscious internal working models which contain generalized information of a negative and persecutory nature about interpersonal relationships with those in authority over her.

Formation of new internal working models

A move from insecure to secure attachments

Research on patients undergoing psychotherapy has shown that one measurable change that takes place is that there is a significant shift from insecure to secure patterns of attachment in the patient population. One tool which has been used to identify such changes is the Adult Attachment Interview (Fonagy 1995: 267). Information, whether in the form of a perception, a memory or a fantasy, becomes meaningful only when it is organized by internal working models which determine the significance of the new information, by providing an implicit pattern into which it can be fitted. Daniel Stern (1985) has described how these patterns develop in childhood, as experiences are collected together into 'schemas of being with' and eventually into RIGs – 'Representations of Interactions that have been Generalized' (Stern 1985). The Adult Attachment Interview reflects the internal working models which organize patterns of attachment.

In analysis, new experiences are constantly registered and stored. If these memories being formed in analysis have a consistent type of content, this store of information may be drawn on to form memories in implicit format, containing information in a schematized and generalized form, reflecting the patterns of experience in the analysis. The formation of new internal working models underpins the shift during therapy from insecure to secure patterns of attachment. The consistency of the analyst's responses to the patient, the sensitive attunement and reflective function of the analyst all contribute to a pattern of relationship which patients can experience as secure and reliable and in which they can become increasingly confident of their own worth. These repeated self–other experiences contribute to the formation of internal working models which contain generalized representations of secure patterns of attachment, derived from the repeated analytic experiences. These internal working models can then organize the perception and experience of new relationships, so contributing to secure patterns of attachment. They are reflected together with their associated secure patterns of attachment in the responses given in the Adult Attachment Interview.

This process may also underpin the experience of 'now' moments which Stern (1994) considers to be crucial points of new experience and change in analysis. A metaphor which might illustrate the emergence of a 'now' moment is that of a set of scales with a gradually increasing weight on one side as new secure internal working models are gradually formed in analysis and a gradually diminishing weight on the other side as old models lose their determining power. A 'now' moment might represent the point at which the scales suddenly shift from the old to the new internal working model. I suggested this metaphor to Daniel Stern at a recent conference and he accepted it as a possible explanation of the relationship between 'now' moments and the gradual underlying change in internal working models (Daniel Stern 2002, personal communication).

One of the key features of borderline personality disorder is that there are multiple but inconsistent internal working models of self–other relationships, leading to marked swings and inconsistency in attitudes, moods and behaviour. Borderline patients seem to have experienced such inconsistent and unpredictable care in childhood that they have not had the opportunity to develop consistent internal working models of relationships. For example, a child may have experienced a parent as being in a very anxious and emotionally needy state on some occasions and then coldly rejecting or possibly violent at other times; this might particularly be the case when a parent has been misusing drugs or alcohol (Fonagy *et al.* 1995; Patrick *et al.* 1994).

Increase in reflective function

One of the purposes of analysis has been defined by Sandler as an 'increase in the capacity for self-observation and self-understanding'

(Sandler and Dreher 1996: 115). In analysis, this frequently requires the capacity to imagine the state of mind and intentions of the people involved in the past events which are being described, in order to render them meaningful (most stories told about the past in analysis are about relationships). The analyst assists the patient in this imaginative process ('What do you think might have been going on in your mother/father's mind when she/he did that?') and so the recollection of autobiographical memories contributes towards the development of reflective function.

The intentions of people involved in a past event, the way their behaviour may illustrate their attitudes both on that and other occasions, form an important part of analytic work. Each time this is explored in the analytic sessions, new narratives are constructed, containing information drawn from the original memory and also including information about the reflective work which has gone on in the analysis. Representations of the communications of both patient and analyst which demonstrate reflective function will be incorporated into these newly constructed narratives which are continuously being formed in the analysis. Representations of the imagined mental functioning of the people involved in the past event will also be incorporated into new internal working models, containing schematized information about self–other relationships as mutually reflective. These models provide the basis for an increase in reflective function which analysis may bring about because they contain representations of mental processes such as thoughts, feelings and intentions (one's own and other people's) as well as representations of physical events and interactions.

A fundamental aspect of reflective function is that it offers a contemporary and more precise account of the achievement of the depressive position, because it describes the information-processing which underpins the capacity to see others as psychologically separate. As Fonagy (1991) has pointed out, even the most psychotic patient is aware that the other person is a physically separate being. It is the ability to recognize psychological separateness which seems a more fragile development, more likely to fail, unless carefully nurtured by parents whose attentive mindfulness can then be internalized and related to intrapsychically in the internal working models which are gradually constructed throughout a child's development.

Change in analysis: a developmental and emergent model

In spite of the difficulties in determining the precise nature of the psychic changes that underpin change at all levels in analysis, it may be possible to draw on the research findings which I have referred to throughout this book to offer an account of the process of change in analysis which integrates the three processes I have explored so far:

- interpretation: enactments and experiences in the analysis are identified as the product of unconscious expectations and the recreation of past patterns of relationship
- the creation of new experiences and hence of new internal working models by means of the interpersonal relationship with the analyst
- the overcoming of a previously inhibited developmental process by the activation of unconscious psychic structures such as image schemas.

The thread which can unite these three aspects of the analytic process is the concept of reflective function. The view that a deficit in reflective function makes a significant contribution to many of the problems and patterns of symptoms that we see in the consulting room has profound implications for our model of the process of change in analysis. It suggests that one of the functions of analysis is to formulate interpretations that demonstrate the analyst's reflective function, to assist in the creation of new internal working models which include representations of reflective function in oneself and others. This can enable psychological separateness and activate the development of previously inhibited psychic structures and the capacity to learn from new experience.

This perspective fundamentally challenges the classical psychoanalytic perspective that the central (and, even, the only) function of analysis is to overcome repression by the interpretation of defences and of unconscious fantasy. In this model, anything else that the analyst adds is suggestion and is not part of the analytic endeavour. However, at the conference held by the *Journal of Analytical Psychology* in Merida, Mexico, in 1999, Owen Renik presented a paper in which he described analytic work, a significant part of which involved the analyst presenting the patient with ideas that he she had not previously considered. Renik's analytic method included the classical analysis of defences and of the unconscious motivations which lay behind those defences, but there were also times when he saw the need to offer a model of his own mind at work in order to help his patient to begin to develop her own.

> If pre-existing thoughts are discovered in analysis, they are of course, the patient's thoughts; whereas if thoughts are newly created in analysis they are necessarily co-authored by patient and analyst . . . very often the most important thing that happens in analysis is that the patient is presented with new thoughts to consider – not thoughts of the patient's which he or she has been motivated to keep unconscious, not memories of pre-verbal experiences which needed verbal presentation in order to reach consciousness but thoughts that the patient has never previously encountered.
>
> (Renik 2000: 7)

Renik goes on to say that, compared with psychoanalysts, analytical psychologists appear to be more comfortable with the idea that the analyst often adds information from his or her own perspective for the patient to consider, rather than only helping the patient to discover in him- or herself thoughts that existed *a priori*.

If we accept that a legitimate part of analytic work involves providing the setting and opportunities for the gradual creation of the patient's capacity for reflective function, then this also has profound implications for technique in clinical practice. Patients whose internal working models lack crucial representations of reflective function are unable to find meaning or symbolic significance in their own actions or those of others. With such patients, the nature of the analyst's interpretations may need to be modified and targeted toward demonstrating the analyst's own reflective function. This can be achieved by the analyst repeatedly showing his or her awareness that all the patient's behaviour is symbolic, that the analyst can find meaning in the patient's non-verbal communications. In other words, the analyst needs to show clearly that he or she relates to the patient as someone with a mind, even when the patient has no sense of his or her own mind at work.

This 'synthetic' or constructive method of analysis is very familiar to Jungians. Jung himself proposed that 'The aim of the constructive method therefore is to elicit from the unconscious product a meaning that relates to the subject's future attitude', a statement that demonstrates his view of the unconscious as a creative contributor to change in analysis (Jung 1921: para. 702). This approach is beautifully exemplified by Fordham (1996) in a passage in which he describes in detail his analytic work with a patient who frequently remained silent for long periods during sessions. Fordham's description shows how his interpretations demonstrate his awareness that there is meaningful communication in the patient's silent behaviour. The concept of reflective function has become prominent only in the 1990s, so it was not a term that Fordham used himself, but the clinical vignette below shows that he used interpretations in a way that could facilitate the development of the patient's reflective function. Fordham described his approach here as a modified version of the classical Jungian technique of amplification. It is modified in the sense that Fordham drew on his own countertransference responses in the form of his spontaneous thoughts and memories, using them as private amplifications which were not communicated to the patient but were drawn on to further his understanding of the patient's unconscious communications to him. These countertransference responses were the result of his own symbolizing capacity, his own reflective function in operation, which could attribute psychological intentionality to the patient's behaviour, when the patient could not see any such meaning himself. Here is Fordham's account of the patient, followed by the clinical vignette:

I will now consider the case of a middle-aged man for whom the uselessness of interpretations was a prominent feature during several years of treatment. When he came to me, after a previous analysis that had lasted nine years, he soon started to mount his attack on analysis with such assertions as 'I've had nine years of useless analysis, what is the use of analysis? It has not done me any good!' He seemed determined to undermine all my efforts to enlighten him by making general statements such as these. Later he became more specific 'What is the use of that?' was one style or 'I don't know what you are talking about!' was another, each theme being elaborated in various ways. Why then did he come with great regularity?

One day this same patient came into the room. He did not look in my direction but settled into the chair and said nothing. He looked half suspicious and half miserable. . . This procedure had been repeated before and I had drawn his attention to what looked like a ritual and had related it to the fact that I regularly filled my pipe at the same time, but no progress had been made except that it was related to his silence and that he needed me to start off the interview even if he did not understand what I meant or even if my interventions were felt to be of no use.

After that I pursued my policy of not knowing. Soon an infant observation came into my mind. A certain baby, from soon after birth, persistently whined and grizzled. In most other respects, his relation to his mother seemed satisfactory. Feeding and nappy changes were well negotiated but the mother never talked to her baby. One day she handed him over to the observer and the infant whined and grizzled as usual till the observer started talking to him – and the whining and grizzling stopped. The mother, usually an observant and sensitive woman, noted what had happened and started talking to her baby; the whining behaviour disappeared though he could not have understood his mother's words. I tried a similar technique with my patients, reflecting that the important thing might be to talk never mind whether he understood.

(Fordham 1996: 193)

This process of integrating and linking is the means by which analysts demonstrate their own reflective function and in doing so assist their patients in developing their own capacity to reflect on and finding meaning in experience. An increasing number of psychoanalysts are moving towards an acceptance of a constructive component in analytic work, recognizing that interpretations cannot focus purely on the overcoming of repression, even though they do not explicitly relate this modification of technique to the idea that they are helping the patient to develop new internal working models which include representations of reflective function. For example, one of the foremost psychoanalytic researchers, Robert Emde (1999), concurs with this view:

Over the course of its history . . . psychoanalytic thinking has increasingly taken into account the importance of the complexities of meaning and of integrative processes – both in practice and in the wider arenas of theory. We are not just analysing, reducing, deconstructing and dying. We are as much concerned with integration, connecting and putting together as we are with analysis.

(Emde 1999: 317)

Another psychoanalyst, Roy Schafer (1999), also challenges the long-established psychoanalytic tradition that the analytic task is to overcome repression:

> [W]e must give up the assumption that what we do when we analyse is *un*cover or *dis*cover or *re*cover what is already there in fully developed form. Instead, we are prepared to assume that there is little or nothing that exists 'out there' in a well-formed manner. It does not exist until it is brought into being and given some kind of shape by an act of naming and characterization within some kind of analytic context and ongoing dialogue. For example, the analytic observer, in dialogue with the analysand, constructs a version of the analysand's representational world and its constructive principles.
>
> (Schafer 1999: 78, original emphases)

Schafer goes on to apply this specifically to the interpretation of enactments. He regards enactments as analytic data that must be regarded as constructions, which the analyst may interpret in a variety of ways, depending on the theoretical model that the analyst relies on. Schafer rejects the idea that it does not matter which theoretical framework an analyst relies on, writing that 'The school of thought provides the theoretical guideline or the interpretative storylines of analytic work' (Shafer 1999: 80).

However, I would suggest that the concept of reflective function offers a meta-theoretical framework which may explain the research finding that the therapeutic effect of analysis does not seem to depend on the theoretical model the analyst uses. This could be the case if what matters in analysis is the fact that the analyst consistently finds meaning in behaviour (enactments) that the patient himself or herself does not yet realize are meaningful. When Michael Fordham attributed psychological intentionality to the patient's polishing his glasses, interpreting this as his wish to see more clearly, he was doing what mothers do with small infants. He was helping the patient to construct an image of himself as a person with desires and intentions, which the analyst could recognize through the patient's actions. It may well be true that the analyst needs a consistent theoretical framework within which to process and find meaning in the patient's communications; on the other hand, for the patient the most fundamental requirement is for an analyst whose theoretical model allows that analyst to see meaning and intentionality in the patient. It probably does not matter too much whether the analyst's interpretations about the patient's intentions are entirely accurate; indeed the analyst's inaccuracies, if not too great, may help patients discover them- selves what their intentions are, just as a baby corrects a mother's small misattunements. Marvin *et al.* (2002) have conducted detailed studies, with rated video tapes, of parents' interactions with their infants as part of a 20-week parent education and psychotherapy intervention designed to shift patterns of attachment in high risk parent–infant dyads (Marvin *et al.* 2002). One of their conclusions is that smooth interactions between parents and their children are often disrupted and need repair, as Bowlby (1969) himself sug- gested. Marvin *et al.* (2002) suggest that it is this ability to repair disruption that is the essence of secure attachment, not the lack of disruptions, and that repair requires a clear understanding and responsiveness to each other's signals. This disruption and repair process in infancy is mirrored in the analytic process in later life, and it depends on the analyst's reflective function, his or her attentiveness and sensitive responsiveness to the feedback from the patient. If the analyst's theoretical framework is one which allows a reasonable degree of understanding of the patient's psychological need for this kind of mutually responsive relationship, then the patient will feel contained. It is the patient's need to be understood, in the sense of being held in mind, which the analyst needs to understand and convey by the nature of his or her interpretations.

The analyst's demonstration of his or her own reflective function seems therefore to be increasingly recognized as a vital part of analytic technique. Even if this is not explicitly stated in attach- ment theory language, I would argue that the attachment theory model of the creation of new internal working models which contain representations of reflective function offers the most com- prehensive and cogent explanation for this aspect of analytic effectiveness, regardless of the theoretical framework which the analyst consciously uses.

Narratives and neurobiology

Daniel Stern's (1985) *The Interpersonal World of the Infant* was one of the first reviews of developmental research to have a major impact on the world of clinical psychoanalytic psychotherapy. Since then an accelerating stream of research has explored the complex relationship between the interpersonal, the emotional and the neurophysiological functioning of both infants and adults. Many of these have begun to investigate the impact of psychotherapy on neural pathways in the brain (Schore 1994; Damasio 1999; LeDoux 1998; Panksepp 1998).

However, the relationship between the information-processing account of change in psychotherapy and the impact of therapy on neurophysiology has, so far, been addressed to only a very limited extent. It is difficult enough to explore the correlation between the subjective world of symbolic meaning with either the information-processing or the neurophysiological model, let alone try to integrate all three levels of explanation. Nevertheless I have argued throughout this book that the psychodynamic understanding of the psyche must be compatible with the current evidence of the cognitive capacities of the human mind and the same applies to neurophysiology.

One key focus for this kind of exploration is the concept of appraisal, which I have briefly described in Chapter 6 on reflective function and which I also suggested plays a key role in maintaining psychic defences by signalling danger. The unconscious meaning that we attribute to events plays a central role in the degree of emotion, pleasant or unpleasant, that those events arouse. Psychoanalytic psychotherapy of all orientations aims to bring about a gradual change in the unconscious meaning attributed to experiences and relationships, both past and present.

LeDoux (1998) places appraisal at the heart of the effect of therapy, writing that 'psychoanalysis, with emphasis on conscious insight and conscious appraisals, may involve the control of the amygdala by explicit knowledge through the temporal lobe memory system and other cortical areas involved in conscious awareness' (LeDoux 1998: 265). However, the connections from the cortical areas to the amygdala are far weaker than the connections from the amygdala to the cortex and this is why it is so easy for us to be swept away by emotion but so difficult to gain conscious control over our emotions. LeDoux's idea that therapy is another way to strengthen the synaptic connections in neural pathways from the cortex that control the amygdala would seem to support Freud's remark that the goal of analysis is that 'where there was id there shall be ego' (Freud 1933: 80). Interpretation and the construction of narratives about the analysand's past and present pattern of relationships would seem to be the main therapeutic tool for strengthening the control that the cortex can exercise over the amygdala.

In contrast, the formation of new internal working models which underpin the emergence of secure attachments and reflective function may relate to other neurophysiological pathways. There would seem to be sound neurophysiological support for Jung's model of the transcendent function as a dialogue between conscious and unconscious processes of appraisal. Allan Schore (2000b: 309) draws on empirical research to support his view that the right hemisphere is predominant in 'performing valence-dependent, automatic, pre-attentive appraisals of emotional facial expressions' and that the orbito-frontal system, in particular, is important in assembling and monitoring relevant past and current experiences, including their affective and social values. Crucially, he extends this appraisal function of the orbito-frontal cortex to underpin reflective function itself, suggesting that the orbito-frontal cortex is particularly involved in theory of mind tasks which have an affective component.

Margaret Wilkinson (2003) offers detailed clinical illustrations to support Schore's view that the prefrontal limbic cortex retains the plastic capacities of early youth and that affectively focused treatment can literally alter the orbito-frontal system. The main vehicle for this is the non-verbal transference-countertransference dynamics which can be considered to be right hemisphere to right hemisphere communications (Wilkinson 2003). These repeated experiences of being with an analyst who is reliable, consistent and empathic are internalized, providing the basis for the gradual creation of new internal working models, which reflect the new patterns of sensitive responsiveness that gradually develop in an intense analytic relationship and store this in the form of 'implicit relational knowledge' (Stern *et al.* 1998). This process reflects the rhythmic dialogue that Sander and others have described so clearly in infancy. Schore summarizes this succinctly:

> The attuned, intuitive clinician, from the first point of contact, is learning the nonverbal moment-to-moment rhythmic structures of the patient's internal states, and is relatively flexibly and fluidly modifying her own behaviour to synchronize with that structure, thereby creating a context for the organization of the therapeutic alliance.
>
> (Schore 2000b: 317)

The role of the self-regulating psyche in the process of change in analysis

So far I have explored the role of interpretation and the slow development of new patterns of relationship and internal working models in analysis. But what of the unique Jungian view of the concept of the psyche as self-regulating and the creative and active role of unconscious processes in counteracting conscious biases? It is rare to find this idea in psychoanalysis and there are key differences from the concept of self organization in attachment theory. In classical psychoanalysis, the unconscious is the reservoir of instinctual impulses and wishes and of the counteracting prohibitions of the superego, whereas in attachment theory the unconscious is formed from the internalization of real experience and the defensive reworking of memories in imagination and fantasy, primarily to protect a positive sense of self.

However, in her remarkable integration of cognitive science and psychoanalysis, Bucci (1997) does suggest an active and constructive role for unconscious imagery:

> [I]t is not that dreams or fantasies are symptoms in the sense of being regressive or pathological forms. Rather, somatic or psychic symptoms may carry out a progressive symbolizing function, in the same sense as dreams and fantasies, where other symbols are not available to be used. Symptoms, like dreams, are fundamentally attempts at symbolizing, healing in the psychic domain, although symptoms may then bring new problems of their own.
>
> (Bucci 1997: 263)

Prior to Bucci, some psychoanalysts have occasionally accorded a creative and constructive role to unconscious processes, and it is extremely interesting to note that they are always those who are familiar with Jung's theories in this respect. Charles Rycroft (1979), for example, wrote:

> dreaming is thus a form of communicating or communing with oneself . . . Put another way, dreaming is a special case of reflexive mental activity, in which the self becomes twofold, one part observing, arguing with, reflecting upon, resisting the

implications of, assenting to, ideas, thoughts, situations imaginatively presented to it by the other.

(Rycroft 1979: 45)

This is very close to Jung's account of the transcendent function, described earlier. However, we do not resolve the problem by simply stating that Jung's model of the psyche defines the unconscious as a co-creator of meaning and symbolism and hence of change in analysis; we still need a developmental and information-processing account of this perspective on psychic change. In Chapter 3, I drew on current research in developmental psychology to support my argument that archetypes are not innate hard-wired structures in the human mind, but instead are best identified as 'image schemas', with primitive meanings, in the form of spatial patterns rather than words, which emerge in the earliest weeks of life and which underpin metaphorical meanings throughout life.

I would argue that the analytic process can activate these image schemas and create the conditions in which a previously inhibited development of the metaphorical extensions of image schemas can begin and so provide the archetypal basis for the process of change in analysis. For example, the image schema or archetype of containment is activated in a safe analytic environment and can become a powerful source of unconscious imagery which can guide the analytic exploration of the experience of containment in all its aspects.

This developmental model of change in analysis, centred on the previously inhibited development of unconscious and primitive patterns of meaning, takes us back full circle to the emergent model of the development of the human mind in infancy that I described in Chapter 3. The process of representational redescription is not limited to the early years of life; it also provides the basis for the gradual emergence of new insight during the analytic process. Image schemas are activated and experienced in implicit ways that initially cannot be described in words. The formation of secure internal working models therefore depends on both the safe and containing experiences with the analyst and the activation of the archetype or image schema of containment. Both external reality and unconscious expectation therefore contribute to the new implicit knowledge contained in internal working models. As the analysis proceeds, a language to describe these implicit psychic patterns can gradually be constructed, through the process of representational redescription, from which explicit knowledge emerges. Narrative competence and reflective function can perhaps therefore be considered as the end-products of the same process that leads to the development of conscious, explicit knowledge, that can be expressed in words, in childhood.

Conclusions

In this chapter I have shown that the process of change in analysis is the end result of a complex interaction of factors. It is a learning process in that new patterns of relationship in analysis are internalized and used to create new unconscious patterns of expectations about future interpersonal experience. It is an integrating process in which representations and unconscious narratives are woven together into a coherent and unified sense of identity. It is also a developmental process in which primitive psychic structures provide a scaffolding that patterns and integrates new experience, allowing the gradual emergence of explicit knowledge and self-awareness.

The art of being an analyst is that of intuitively knowing when to use each of the therapeutic tools of interpretation, containment or the co-construction of new narratives, not one of which is sufficient on its own.

Chapter 8

Conclusions

Science and symbols

I hope that those readers who have stayed with me as far as this final chapter will be clearer about the course that psychoanalysis and analytical psychology must steer between two opposing dangers. There is the danger of a scientific and deterministic imperialism which attempts to reduce the complexity of the human psyche to explanation in terms of one unified theory. Dupré (2001) suggests that evolutionary psychology is one such example, and writes in scathing terms of this approach, in relation to Stephen Pinker's (1997) *How the Mind Works*:

> The view that is presented therein, that the mind is a computer programmed by natural selection in the Stone Age, is as reductive and simplistic an approach to its topic as anyone is likely seriously to propose, and is as lacking in serious insight into the human condition as such an attempt is likely to prove.
> (Dupré 2001: 184)

Dupré argues that, in contrast to this kind of highly specialized approach that mistakenly includes phenomena which are outside its range of explanation, we need to learn to move between different disciplines:

> If a subject matter can only be understood from simultaneous attention to a variety of perspectives, then knowledge of a subject matter will require access to diverse bodies of information. And perhaps part of what amounts to wisdom is the ability to know what kinds of information or knowledge are needed in application to a particular case.
> (Dupré 2001: 186)

However, if the scientific paradigm is discarded altogether, the pluralism that Dupré proposes can slide too easily into a post-modern multiplicity of theoretical narratives which have no connection with the growing body of empirical research in other disciplines about the way the mind takes in and organizes information. Anthony Stevens (2002) focuses on this danger, stating:

> My position is that there exists a place for pluralism and contextualization, but that Jungian psychology will destroy itself if it does not recognize certain basic principles, which are not 'beliefs' or 'fictions', but hypotheses which have passed certain empirical tests.
>
> (Stevens 2002: 349)

Stevens suggests that his successful demolition of Richard Noll's (1994) attack on Jung's theory of archetypes was founded on the scientific evidence which supports Jung's model. Stevens concludes that 'to ignore or dismiss the biological contribution to this evidence, as some Jungians seem prepared to do, is to squander a priceless asset' (Stevens 2002: 350). This book is my contribution to the thorough examination of the models of the mind which analysts need to undertake in the light of available empirical evidence and I know from my own conversation with Stevens that he entirely agrees that a proper debate about these differences of viewpoint plays a key role in the scientific endeavour. While I share his view that the scientific approach is a vital tool with which to examine the theory and practice of analytical psychology, I consider that there is an accumulating body of empirical evidence which leads to rather different conclusions about the human psyche from those drawn by Stevens. I have reviewed the research which underpins my view that complex mental imagery and ideation cannot be encoded genetically and that attempts to argue that what we inherit is a potential for imagery with specific archetypal and symbolic significance is also doomed to failure.

As I stated in Chapter 3, the essence of the problem is twofold; first, the human genome contains only 30,000 genes and this is totally inadequate for a model in which 'external events are already "planned for"' in the sense that the various possibilities are genetically built into the programme so as to permit the organism, by using its cognitive apparatus, to select that which is 'best suited to the environmental circumstances prevailing at any moment'

(Stevens 2002: 61). Even the complex human genome can encode only a few automatic behaviour patterns which are essential for survival, like the first moves in a chess game; after that the number of possible moves becomes too vast for even a chess grand-master to anticipate, and the number of genes required to store all that potential information does not exist in any living creature.

The second problem with the view that the archetype-as-such is genetically encoded is linked to the first issue. A response to certain physical patterns, such as the arrangement of hair, eyes, nose and mouth in the face, may be genetically encoded, but this is a behavioural response to a physical stimulus. The symbolic significance of faces is not and could not be genetically stored. The consistent problem with Stevens's argument is his reliance on instinctually based behaviour patterns in animals to support his view that the archetype-as-such is inherited. He uses the example of nest building in birds to argue that

> a bird must have some kind of 'image' of what a completed nest should be like. The image may or may not be conscious, but clearly there is some central mechanism that 'knows' how a nest should be built and which coordinates the energies of the bird as it builds it.
>
> (Stevens 2002: 60)

Although Stevens argues that his model is compatible with evolutionary psychology, this view would seem to be in direct contradiction to Dennett's (1995) unequivocal statement that this kind of complex instinctive pattern of behaviour is the result of a sequence of 'algorithms', each of which is automatically triggered by certain environmental stimuli. There is no central plan, only a cascade of separate automatic routines, largely controlled by the subcortex, which have evolved by natural selection, and which create sequences of behaviour that can deceive the observer into believing there is a coordinating mechanism when there is not, as I showed in Chapter 3.

It is a very different matter when we come to the infinitely variable ideation and symbolic imagery which depends on the functioning of the human cortex. Symbolic meaning depends on the process of evaluation and comparison of experiences with each other – in other words it depends on information from the real world. Jean Mandler (1998) has convincingly shown that from about the age of 6 months, the human infant develops the capacity for perceptual analysis and so for the earliest forms of concept formation. The human brain sorts information, finding similarities and differences which constitute the basis of symbolization, and this kind of categorization develops through repeated experience and is not innate. The concept of mother, for example, is built up from the multitude of daily experiences in a small child's life – it is not and cannot be inherited and to suggest that it can be is to fall straight into the discredited Lamarckian trap.

The developmental model of the mind which runs like a thread through this book is that emergence provides the key to our attempts to reconcile biology with psyche. Emergence is a concept that overcomes the problems of finding an accurate definition of archetypes that Jung struggled with all his life and which still plagues analytical psychologists to this day. The model that I have offered here is that mind and meaning are constructed on the foundation stones of brain, instinct and perception. Meaning emerges out of the way in which the brain organizes the mass of information presented to it every second, even though the starting point for this process is a few instinctual patterns of behaviour which, unlike symbolic mental content, are fixed sub-cortical routines, which can be hard-wired and inherited genetically.

The role of genes is to act as catalysts, kick-starting the process by activating a few automatic patterns of behaviour, such as the attentional mechanism 'Conspec' described in Chapter 3. The constant process of perceptual analysis that Jean Mandler delineated is then set in motion, leading to the formation of the earliest psychic constructs, image schemas. I suggest that these offer us the most internally consistent model for archetypes, meeting the requirements that archetypes should be part of the collective human psyche, without innate imagery in themselves, but giving rise to regularly repeated patterns of meaning. They are the nuclei of meaning which emerge with total predictability in the earliest weeks of human development, with one essential proviso – the environment during those early weeks has to be the species-typical environment and the essential feature of this is a loving, nurturing and attentive parent. The lack of that essential relationship has a devastating effect on human development; emotionally neglected infants and children fail to thrive, fall ill, their intellectual and emotional development is profoundly impaired and they have a much higher mortality rate than normal (Karen 1998: 13–25). I suggested in Chapter 3 that this impairment could also lead to a distorted development of image schemas.

Complex symbolic imagery is constructed around image schema nuclei through the process of representational redescription as Karmiloff-Smith (1992) suggests, a model which provides an information-processing account of the cycle of deintegration and reintegration delineated by Michael Fordham (1985). The essential feature of this process is a constant comparison between the mass of new information absorbed through the senses every minute and the patterns of core meaning which are slowly built up in the psyche, the general 'mental models' described by Johnson-Laird (1991) and the more specific 'internal working models' of personal identity and relationship described by John Bowlby (1973).

This is a two-way process; regularly repeated patterns of experience become internalized and so form part of our psychic structure as mental models and these in turn structure our perception of the world, determining how we interpret what we see, hear and feel. The repeated patterns of daily experience gradually build up into a generalized schema which forms the basis, for example, for the symbolic concept of mother or father. The unique contribution that attachment theory makes to our understanding of this process is that it acts as a bridge between the scientific and the symbolic, identifying the interpersonal processes which form the foundation for the construction of meaning in the mind. It places emotion at the heart of the developmental process, a view which is gaining increasing support from neurophysiological research which demonstrates that brain development crucially depends on experience, with the vast majority of the critical structural organization taking place in childhood (Perry 1999: 11).

Awareness of the symbolic meaning of experiences is a two-edged sword. Instead of providing the sense of depth and richness which we need for life to be satisfying and purposeful, meaning can become traumatic and terrifying. Clinical work demonstrates time and again the intense distress that a small child feels if he or she is unloved, neglected or treated with hostility and cruelty. The child's fundamental sense of his or her worth as a human being is threatened and this narcissistic wound activates powerful defences which operate to lessen this distress, but at the price of a diminished capacity for secure and trusting intimacy. Defensive fantasies are elaborated unconsciously to explain trauma in terms that pose less threat to a person's very sense of identity – it seems to be unbearable to be treated as an object and for one's essential subjectivity to be seen as of no importance. Habitual psychological trauma of this kind may lead to the ultimate defence, the suppression of the meaning-making process itself, since reflective function leads to the child's awareness of intentional cruelty in the minds of those very people that he or she loves and needs.

As Stevens (2002) says, the area where two disciplines meet is often charged with the most energy and the most excitement. I have taken up his challenge that constructivism must give way to evolutionary concepts in the study of the mind and instead I suggest that contructionism and biology can be reconciled in a model of the mind as self-organizing. An emergent view of the development of symbolic meaning has grown out of attachment theory, which is both constructionist and biological, and out of the research of developmental psychologists who firmly embed the emergence of meaning in bodily experience. I hope that the most original contribution of this book has been to link the two approaches together, to show that the construction of unconscious complex representational meaning is founded and crucially depends on the early emergence of image schemas which construct physical patterns of meaning of the world around the small infant.

This approach does nothing less than overcome the Cartesian dualism that has plagued philosophy and psychology for centuries. Descartes thought that the world is divided into physical and mental substances and argued that the only thing we can know with certainty is not our bodies but our minds. Johnson offers a revolutionary solution to this 'ontological gulf between mind and body, reason and sensation' by suggesting that the body does indeed play a crucial role in human reasoning (Johnson 1987: xxvi). He suggests that imaginative projection is the process by which bodily experience works its way up into the mind. Image schemas – embodied patterns of imagination – determine and constrain the ways in which we connect things together in our minds.

I think that Jung also struggled to find a solution to Cartesian dualism and his concept of archetypes was, in many respects, a remarkable anticipation of some of the key features of the 'bodily basis of meaning, imagination and reason' offered by Johnson (1987).

The imaginative world, in all its richness, is the thread that links psyche and soma and that weaves archetypes, attachment and analysis together into a synthesis of the developmental, emergent and introjective aspects of the human mind. I hope that the reader has been able to follow that thread with me through this book.

Bibliography

Affeld-Niemayer, P. (1995) 'Trauma and symbol: instinct and reality perception in therapeutic work with victims of incest', *Journal of Analytical Psychology*, 40(1): 23–40.

Ainsworth, M., Blehar, M., Waters, E. and Wall, S. (1978) *Patterns of Attachment: Assessed in the Strange Situation and at Home*, Hillsdale, NJ: Erlbaum.

American Psychiatric Association (APA) (1994) *Diagnostic and Statistical Manual of Mental Disorders*, 4th edn (DSM-IV), Washington, DC: APA.

Arlow, J. (1996) 'The concept of psychic reality: how useful?', *International Journal of Psychoanalysis*, 77(4): 659–66.

Astor, J. (1995) *Michael Fordham: Innovations in Analytical Psychology*, London and New York: Routledge.

Baddeley, A.D. and Hitch, G. (1974) 'Working memory', in G.H. Bower (ed.) *The Psychology of Learning and Motivation*, vol. 8, New York: Academic Press.

Bailey, K. (2000) 'Evolution, kinship and psychotherapy: promoting psychological health through human relationship', in P. Gilbert and K. Bailey (eds) *Genes on the Couch. Explorations in Evolutionary Psychotherapy*, Hove: Brunner-Routledge.

Barkow, J.H., Cosmides, J. and Tooby, L. (1992) *The Adapted Mind: Evolutionary Psychology and the Generation of Culture*, New York and Oxford: Oxford University Press.

Baron-Cohen, S. (1988) 'Social and pragmatic deficits in autism: cognitive or affective?', *Journal of Autism and Developmental Disorders*, 18: 379–402.

Bartlett, F.C. (1932) *Remembering*, Cambridge: Cambridge University Press.

Beck, L. (1998) *Cognitive Development in Infancy and Toddlerhood*, Boston, MA: Allyn and Bacon.

Bion, W.R. (1959) 'Attacks on linking', *International Journal of Psychoanalysis*, 40: 308–15.
—— (1962) *Learning from Experience*, London: Heinemann.
Bishop, P. (1999) *Jung in Contexts*, London and New York: Routledge.
—— (2000) *Synchronicity and Intellectual Intuition in Kant, Swedenborg and Jung*, New York: Edwin Mellen.
Blasco, D.G. and Merski, D.W. (1998) 'Haiku poetry and metaphorical thought: an invitation to interdisciplinary study', *Creativity Research Journal*, 11(1): 39–46.
Blaxton, T.A. (1989) 'Investigating dissociations among memory measures: support for a transfer-appropriate processing framework', *Journal of Experimental Psychology: Learning, Memory and Cognition*, 15: 657–68.
Bovensiepen, G. (2002) 'Symbolic attitude and reverie: problems of symbolization in children and adolescents', *Journal of Analytical Psychology*, 47(2): 241–58.
Bowlby, J. (1969) *Attachment and Loss*, vol. 1, *Attachment*, London: Hogarth Press.
—— (1973) *Attachment and Loss*, vol. 2, *Separation: Anxiety and Anger*, London: Hogarth Press and the Institute of Psychoanalysis.
—— (1979) *The Making and Breaking of Affectional Bonds*, London: Tavistock.
—— (1980) *Attachment and Loss*, vol. 3, *Loss: Sadness and Depression*, London: Hogarth Press and the Institute of Psychoanalysis.
—— (1988) *A Secure Base: Clinical Applications of Attachment Theory*, London: Routledge.
Bretherton, I. (1985) 'Attachment theory: retrospect and prospect', in I. Bretherton and E. Waters (eds) *Growing Points in Attachment Theory and Research, Monographs of the Society for Research in Child Development*, 50 (1–2, serial no. 209): 3–38.
—— (1995) 'The origins of attachment theory', in S. Goldberg, R. Muir and J. Kerr (eds) *Attachment Theory Social: Developmental and Clinical Perspectives*, Hillsdale, NJ and London: Analytic Press.
—— (1999) 'Updating the "internal working model": bridging the transmission gap', *Attachment and Human Development*, 1(3): 343–57.
Bretherton, I. and Munholland, K. (1999) 'Internal working models in attachment relationships: a construct revisited', in J. Cassidy and P. Shaver (eds) *Handbook of Attachment: Theory, Research and Clinical Applications*, New York and London: Guilford Press.
Brewin, C., Dalgleish, T. and Joseph, S. (1996) 'A dual representation theory of post-traumatic stress disorder', *Psychological Review*, 103(4): 670–86.
Brooke, R. (1991) *Jung and Phenomenology*, London and New York: Routledge.

Broussard, E. (1970) 'Maternal perception of the neonate as related to development', *Child Psychiatry and Human Development*, 1: 16–25.

Brown, G.W. and Harris, T. (1978) *Social Origins of Depression*, London: Tavistock.

Bruner, J.S. (1986) *Actual Minds, Possible Worlds*, Cambridge, MA: Harvard University Press.

Bucci, W. (1997) *Psychoanalysis and Cognitive Science, A Multiple Code Theory*, New York and London: Guilford Press.

Cain, A.C. and Fast, I. (1972) 'Children's disturbed reactions to parent suicide', in A.C. Cain (ed.) *Survivors of Suicide*, Springfield, IL: Charles C. Thomas.

Campos, J. *et al.* (1983) 'Socioemotional development' in P. Mussen (ed.) *Handbook of Child Psychology*, vol II, New York: John Wiley.

Carrette, J.R. (1994) 'The language of archetypes: a conspiracy in psychological theory', *Harvest*, 40: 168–93.

Casement, A. (2001) *Carl Gustav Jung*, London: Sage.

Cassidy, J. (2001) 'Truth, lies and intimacy: an attachment perspective', *Attachment and Human Development*, 3(2): 121–55.

Churchland, P. (1988) 'Reduction and the neurobiological basis of consciousness', in A.E. Marcel and E. Bisiach (eds) *Consciousness in Contemporary Science*, Oxford: Clarendon Press.

Clyman, R. (1991) 'The procedural organization of emotions: a contribution from cognitive science to the psychoanalytic theory of therapeutic action', *Journal of the American Psychoanalytic Association*, 39 (supplement): 349–82.

Cole-Detke, H. and Kobak, R. (1996) 'Attachment processes in eating disorder and depression', *Journal of Consulting and Clinical Psychology*, 64(2): 282–90.

Conway, M. (1990) 'Conceptual representation of emotions: the role of autobiographical memories', in K.J.G. Gilhooly, M.T.G. Keane, R.H. Logie and G. Erdos (eds) *Lines of Thinking*, vol. 2, London: John Wiley.

Cortina, M. (2003) 'Defensive processes, emotions and internal working models. A perspective from attachment theory and contemporary models of the mind', in M. Cortina and M. Marrone (eds) *Attachment Theory and the Psychoanalytic Process*, London: Whurr Publishers.

Damasio, A. (1999) *The Feeling of What Happens*, London: William Heinemann.

Dawkins, R. (1998) *Unweaving the Rainbow*, London: Allen Lane/The Penguin Press.

Dennett, D. (1995) *Darwin's Dangerous Idea: Evolution and the Meanings of Life*, London: Allen Lane/The Penguin Press.

De Voogd, S. (1984) 'Fantasy versus fiction: Jung's Kantianism appraised', in R. Papadopoulos and G. Saayman (eds) *Jung in Modern Perspective*, London: Wildwood House.

Douglas, C. (1997) 'The historical context of analytical psychology', in P. Young-Eisendrath and T. Dawson (eds) *The Cambridge Companion to Jung*, Cambridge: Cambridge University Press.

Dozier, M., Lomax, L., Tyrrell, C.L. and Lee, S.W. (2001) 'The challenge of treatment for clients with dismissing states of mind', *Attachment and Human Development*, 3(1): 31–61.

Dreher, A.-U. (2000) *Foundations for Conceptual Research in Psycho-analysis*, trans. E. Ristl, London and New York: Karnac.

Dupré, J. (2001) *Human Nature and the Limits of Science*, Oxford: Clarendon Press.

Eagle, M. (1995) 'The developmental perspectives of attachment and psychoanalytic theory', in S. Goldberg, R. Muir and J. Kerr (eds) *Attachment Theory: Social, Developmental and Clinical Perspectives*, Hillsdale, NJ and London: Analytic Press.

Edelman, G. (1994 [1992]) *Bright Air, Brilliant Fire: On the Matter of the Mind*, London: Penguin, originally published by Basic Books.

Edelman, G. and Tononi, G. (2000) *Consciousness: How Matter Becomes Imagination*, London: Allen Lane/The Penguin Press.

Ekstrom, S. (2002) 'A cacophony of theories: contributions towards a story-based understanding of analytic treatments', *Journal of Analytical Psychology*, 47(3): 339–58.

Eliot, T.S. (1935) 'Burnt Norton', in *Collected Poems 1909–1962*. Published in 1963. London: Faber & Faber.

Ellenberger, H.F. (1970) *The Discovery of the Unconscious: The History and Evolution of Dynamic Psychiatry*, London: Allen Lane/The Penguin Press.

Elman, J.L., Bates, E.A., Johnson, M.H., Karmiloff-Smith, A., Parisi, D. and Plunkett, K. (1999) *Rethinking Innateness: A Connectionist Perspective on Development*, Cambridge, MA and London: MIT Press.

Emde, R. (1992) 'Individual meaning and increasing complexity: contributions of Sigmund Freud and René Spitz to developmental psychology', *Developmental Psychology*, 28: 347–59.

—— (1999) 'Moving ahead: integrating influences of affective processes for development and for psychoanalysis', *International Journal of Psycho-analysis*, 80(2): 317–40.

Erdelyi, M.H. (1995) 'Repression, reconstruction and defence', in J. Singer (ed.) *Repression and Dissociation: Implications for Personality Theory, Psychopathology and Health*, Chicago and London: University of Chicago Press.

Fabre, J.H. (1916) *The Life of the Caterpillar*, trans. A.T. de Mattos, New York: Dodd, Mead & Co.

Fairbairn, W.R.D. (1941) 'A revised psychopathology of the psychoses and psychoneuroses', in *Psychoanalytic Studies of the Personality*, London: Tavistock.

Ferenczi, S. (1933) 'Confusion of tongues between the adults and the children', in *Final Contributions to the Problems and Methods of Psychoanalysis*, London: Hogarth Press.

Fodor, J. (1983) *The Modularity of Mind*, Cambridge, MA: MIT Press.

Fonagy, P. (1991) 'Thinking about thinking: some clinical and theoretical considerations in the treatment of a borderline patient', *International Journal of Psychoanalysis*, 72(4): 639–56.

—— (1995) 'Psychoanalytic and empirical approaches to developmental psychopathology: an object-relations perspective', in T. Shapiro and R.N. Emde (eds) *Research in Psychoanalysis: Process, Development, Outcome*, Madison, CT: International Universities Press.

—— (1997) 'Perspectives on the recovered memories debate', in J. Sandler and P. Fonagy (eds) *Recovered Memories of Abuse: True or False?* London: Karnac.

—— (1999a) 'Memory and therapeutic action', *International Journal of Psychoanalysis*, 80(2): 215–24.

—— (1999b) 'Psychoanalysis and attachment theory', in J. Cassidy and P. Shaver (eds) *Handbook of Attachment: Theory, Research and Clinical Applications*, New York and London: Guilford Press.

—— (2001) *Attachment Theory and Psychoanalysis*, New York: Other Press.

Fonagy, P. and Tallindini-Shallice, M. (1993) 'Problems of psychoanalytic research in practice', *Bulletin of the Anna Freud Centre*, 16(1): 5–22.

Fonagy, P. and Target, M. (1997) 'Perspectives in the recovered memories debate', in J. Sandler and P. Fonagy (eds) *Recovered Memories of Abuse: True or False?*, London: Karnac.

Fonagy, P., Steele, H., Moran, G., Steele, M. and Higgit, A. (1991) 'The capacity for understanding mental states: the reflective self in parent and child and its significance for security of attachment', *Infant Mental Health Journal*, 13: 200–17.

Fonagy, P., Steele, M., Steele, H., Leigh, T., Kennedy, R., Mattoon, G. and Target, M. (1995) 'Attachment, the reflective self, and borderline states', in S. Goldberg, R. Muir and J. Kerr (eds) *Attachment Theory: Social, Developmental and Clinical Perspectives*, Hillsdale, NJ and London: Analytic Press.

Fordham, M. (1957) *New Developments in Analytical Psychology*, London: Routledge and Kegan Paul.

—— (1963) 'The empirical foundation and theories of the self in Jung's works', in *Analytical Psychology: A Modern Science*, Library of Analytical Psychology, vol. 1, London: William Heinemann.

—— (1969) *Children as Individuals: An Analytical Psychologist's Study of Child Development*, London: Hodder and Stoughton.

—— (1985) *Explorations into the Self*, Library of Analytical Psychology, vol. 7, London: Academic Press.

Fordham, M. (1985[1947]) 'Defences of the self', in *Explorations into the Self*, Library of Analytical Psychology, vol, 7. London: Academic Press, originally published in *Journal of Analytical Psychology*, 19(2).

—— (1989) 'The infant's reach', *Psychological Perspectives*, 21: 58–76.

—— (1996) 'The supposed limits of interpretation', in S. Shamdasani (ed.) *Analyst–Patient Interaction: Collected Papers on Technique*, London: Routledge.

Fosshage, J. (2002) 'A relational self psychological perspective', *Journal of Analytical Psychology*, 47(1): 67–82.

Fox, N., Kagan, J. and Weiskopf, S. (1979) 'The growth of memory during infancy', *Genetic Psychology Monographs*, 99: 91–130.

Fraiberg, S., Adelson, E. and Shapiro, V. (1975) 'Ghosts in the nursery: a psychoanalytic approach to the problem of impaired infant–mother relationships', *Journal of the American Academy of Child Psychiatry*, 14: 387–422.

Frayley, R.C. and Shaver, P.R. (1999) 'Loss and bereavement: attachment theory and recent controversies concerning "grief work" and the nature of detachment', in J. Cassidy and P. Shaver (eds) *Handbook of Attachment: Theory, Research and Clinical Applications*, New York and London: Guilford Press.

Freeman, C.P.L. (1994) 'Personality disorders', in R.E. Kendall and A.K. Zealley (eds) *Companion to Psychiatric Studies*, 5th edn, Edinburgh: Churchill Livingstone.

Freud, S. (1895) 'Project for a scientific psychology', *Standard Edition*, vol. 1, London: Hogarth Press.

—— (1905) 'Three Essays on Sexuality', *Standard Edition*, vol. 7, London: Hogarth Press.

—— (1915) 'Repression', *Standard Edition*, vol. 14, London: Hogarth Press.

—— (1923) 'The Ego and the Id', *Standard Edition*, vol. 19, London: Hogarth Press.

—— (1933) 'New introductory lectures', *Standard Edition*, vol. 22, London: Hogarth Press.

—— (1940[1938]) 'An Outline of Psychoanalysis', *Standard Edition*, vol. 23, London: Hogarth Press.

Freud, S. and Breuer, J. (1893) 'On the psychical mechanism of hysterical phenomena: preliminary communication', *Studies on Hysteria, Standard Edition*, vol. 2, London: Hogarth Press.

Frey-Rohn, L. (1974) *From Freud to Jung: A Comparative Study of the Psychology of the Unconscious*, New York: C.G. Jung Foundation for Analytical Psychology.

Garwood, A. (1996) 'The Holocaust and the power of powerlessness: survivor guilt an unhealed wound', *British Journal of Psychotherapy*, 13(2): 243–58.

Gergely, G. (1992) 'Developmental reconstructions: infancy from the point of view of psychoanalysis and developmental psychology', *Psychoanalysis and Contemporary Thought*, 15(1): 3–56.

Gergely, G. and Watson, J. (1996) 'The social biofeedback model of parental affective mirroring', *International Journal of Psychoanalysis*, 77: 1181–212.

Gergely, G., Nadasy, Z., Csibra, G. and Biro, S. (1995) 'Taking the intentional stance at 12 months of age', *Cognition*, 56: 165–93.

Gilbert, P. (1995) 'Biopsychological approaches and evolutionary theory as aids to integration in clinical psychology and psychotherapy', *Clinical Psychology and Psychotherapy*, 2(3): 135–56.

Goldberg, S. (2000) *Attachment and Human Development*, London: Arnold.

Gordon, R. (1993) *Bridges: Metaphor for Psychic Processes*, London: Karnac.

Green, A. (2001) 'Science and science fiction', in J. Sandler, A-M. Sandler and R. Davies (eds) *Clinical and Observational Psychoanalytic Research*, London: Karnac.

Greenberg, J.R. and Mitchell, S.A. (1983) *Object Relations in Psychoanalytic Theory*, Cambridge, MA and London: Harvard University Press.

Grossman, K. (1995) 'The evolution and history of attachment research', in S. Goldberg, R. Muir and J. Kerr (eds) *Attachment Theory: Social, Developmental and Clinical Perspectives*, Hillsdale, NJ and London: Analytic Press.

Gunter, P.A.Y. (1999) 'Bergson and Jung', in P. Bishop (ed.) *Jung in Contexts: A Reader*, London: Routledge.

Hamann, S.B. (1990) 'Level-of-processing effects in conceptually driven implicit tasks', *Journal of Experimental Psychology: Learning, Memory and Cognition*, 16: 970–7.

Hamilton, V. (1996) *The Analyst's Preconscious*, Hillsdale, NJ and London: Analytic Press.

Harlow, H. (1958) 'The nature of love', *American Psychologist*, 13: 673–85.

Hauke, C. (2000) *Jung and the Postmodern: The Interpretation of Realities*, London and Philadelphia, PA: Routledge.

Haule, J. (1999) 'From somnambulism to archetypes: the French roots of Jung's split with Freud', in P. Bishop (ed.) *Jung in Contexts*, London and New York: Routledge.

Hayman, R. (1999) *A Life of Jung*, London: Bloomsbury.

Hinshelwood, R. (1989) *A Dictionary of Kleinian Thought*, London: Free Association.

Hogenson, G. (2001) 'The Baldwin effect: a neglected influence on C.G. Jung's evolutionary thinking', *Journal of Analytical Psychology*, 46(4): 591–612.

Holmes, J. (1993) *John Bowlby and Attachment Theory*, London and New York: Routledge.

—— (2001) *The Search for the Secure Base*, Hove: Brunner-Routledge.

Homans, P. (1979) *Jung in Context: Modernity and the Making of a Psychology*, Chicago: University of Chicago Press.

Isaacs, S. (1948) 'On the nature and function of phantasy', *International Journal of Psychoanalysis*, 29: 73–97; republished (1952) in M. Klein, P. Heimann, S. Isaacs and J. Riviere (eds) *Developments in Psychoanalysis*, London: Hogarth Press.

Jacobi, J. (1959) *Complex/Archetype/Symbol in the Psychology of C.G. Jung*, New York: Bollingen Series Pantheon.

Jacobs, T.J. (2002) 'Response to the *Journal of Analytical Psychology*'s questionnaire', 47(1): 17–34.

Jacoby, M. (1999) *Jungian Psychotherapy and Contemporary Infant Research: Basic Patterns of Emotional Exchange*, London and New York: Routledge.

Jaffe, J., Beebe, B., Feldstein, S., Crown, C. and Jasnow, M.D. (2001) 'Rhythms of dialogue in infancy: coordinated timing in development', *Monographs of the Society for Research in Child Development*, serial no. 265, 66, 2, series editor W.F. Overton. Boston, MA: Blackwell.

Janet, P. (1925[1919]) *Psychological Healing*, vols 1–2, New York: Macmillan; original publication *Les Medications Psychologiques*, vols 1–3, Paris: Alcan.

Jarrett, J.L. (1999) 'Schopenhauer and Jung', in P. Bishop (ed.) *Jung in Contexts*, London and New York: Routledge.

Johnson, M. (1987) *The Body in the Mind: The Bodily Basis of Meaning, Imagination and Reason*, Chicago and London: University of Chicago Press.

Johnson, M.H. and Morton, J. (1991) *Biology and Cognitive Development: The Case of Face Recognition*, Oxford: Blackwell.

Johnson-Laird, P.N. (1991) 'Mental models', in M.I. Posner (ed.) *Foundations in Cognitive Science*, Cambridge, MA and London: MIT Press.

Jung, C.G. (1957–79) *The Collected Works of C.G. Jung*, H. Read, M. Fordham, G. Adler and W. McGuire (eds), trans. R.F.C. Hull, London: Routledge & Kegan Paul. Hereafter called *Collected Works*.

—— (1913) 'The theory of psychoanalysis', *Collected Works*, vol. 4.

—— (1916) 'Psychoanalysis and neurosis', *Collected Works*, vol. 4.

—— (1918) 'The role of the unconscious', *Collected Works*, vol. 10.

—— (1919) 'Instinct and the unconscious', *Collected Works*, vol. 8.

—— (1920) 'Foreword to Evans: "The problem of the nervous child"', *Collected Works*, vol. 18.

—— (1921) 'Definitions', *Collected Works*, vol. 6.

—— (1934) 'A review of the complex theory', *Collected Works*, vol. 8.

Jung, C.G. (1935) 'Tavistock Lecture II', *Collected Works*, vol. 18.
—— (1936) 'Psychological typology', *Collected Works*, vol. 6.
—— (1939) 'Conscious, unconscious and individuation', *Collected Works*, vol. 9i.
—— (1944) 'Introduction to the religious and psychological problems of alchemy', *Collected Works*, vol. 12.
—— (1946) 'The psychology of the transference', *Collected Works*, vol. 16.
—— (1948[1942]) 'A psychological approach to the dogma of the Trinity', *Collected Works*, vol. 11.
—— 1951) 'Fundamental questions of psychotherapy', *Collected Works*, vol. 16.
—— (1954[1934]) 'Archetypes of the collective unconscious', *Collected Works*, vol. 9i.
—— (1954[1936]) 'Concerning the archetypes', *Collected Works*, vol. 9i.
—— (1954[1938]) 'Psychological aspects of the mother archetype', *Collected Works*, vol. 9i.
—— (1954[1946]) 'On the nature of the psyche', *Collected Works*, vol. 8.
—— (1954[1947]) 'On the nature of the psyche', *Collected Works*, vol. 8.
—— (1955) 'Foreword to Harding: "Woman's mysteries"', *Collected Works*, vol. 18.
—— (1956) 'Symbols of transformation', *Collected Works*, vol. 5.
—— (1957[1916]) 'The transcendent function', *Collected Works*, vol. 8.
—— (1960[1934]) 'A review of the complex theory', *Collected Works*, vol. 8.
—— (1963) *C.G. Jung Letters*, vol. 2. Eds. G. Adler and A. Jaffe, Princeton, NJ: Princeton University Press.
—— (1967) 'The detachment of consciousness from the object', *Collected Works*, vol. 13.
Kalsched, D. (1996) *The Inner World of Trauma: Archetypal Defenses of the Personal Spirit*, London and New York: Routledge.
—— (2002) 'Response to Gustav Bovensiepen', *Journal of Analytical Psychology*, 47(2): 259–64.
—— (2003) 'Daimonic elements in early trauma', *Journal of Analytical Psychology*.
Karen, R. (1998) *Becoming Attached: First Relationships and How They Shape our Capacity to Love*, New York and Oxford: Oxford University Press.
Karmiloff-Smith, A. (1992) *Beyond Modularity: A Developmental Perspective on Cognitive Science*, Cambridge, MA: MIT Press.
Kernberg, O. (1988) 'Object relations theory in clinical practice', *Psychoanalytic Quarterly*, 57: 481–504.
Kerz-Kuhling, I. (1996) 'The validation of psychoanalytic hypotheses', *International Journal of Psychoanalysis*, 77(2): 275–90.
Kihlstrom, J.F. and Hoyt, I.P. (1990) 'Repression, dissociation and

hypnosis', in J. Singer (ed.) *Repression and Dissociation: Implications for Personality Theory, Psychopathology and Health*, Chicago: University of Chicago Press.

Kirsch, T. (2001) *The Jungians: A Comparative and Historical Perspective*, London and Philadelphia, PA: Routledge.

Klein, M. (1927) 'Symposium on child-analysis', in *Love, Guilt and Reparation and Other Works: The Writings of Melanie Klein*, vol. 1, London: Hogarth Press.

—— (1932) 'The psychoanalysis of children', in *The Writings of Melanie Klein*, vol. 2, London: Hogarth Press.

—— (1933) 'The early development of conscience in the child', in *Love, Guilt and Reparation and Other Works: The Writings of Melanie Klein*, vol. 1, London: Hogarth Press.

—— (1946) 'Notes on some schizoid mechanisms', in *The Writings of Melanie Klein*, vol. 3, London: Hogarth Press.

—— (1952) 'Some theoretical conclusions regarding the emotional life of the infant', in *The Writings of Melanie Klein*, vol. 3, London: Hogarth Press.

Knox, J. (1997) 'Internal objects: a theoretical analysis of Jungian and Kleinian models', *Journal of Analytical Psychology*, 42(4): 653–66.

—— (1999) 'The relevance of attachment theory to a contemporary Jungian view of the internal world: internal working models, implicit memory and internal objects', *Journal of Analytical Psychology*, 44(4): 511–30.

Kobak, R. (1999) 'The emotional dynamics of disruptions in attachment relationships', in J. Cassidy and P. Shaver (eds) *Handbook of Attachment: Theory, Research and Clinical Applications*, New York and London: Guilford Press.

Kohut, H. (1972) 'Thoughts on narcissism and narcissistic rage', *Psychoanalytic Study of the Child*, 27: 360–400.

—— (1984) *How Does Analysis Cure?*, edited by A. Goldberg and P. Stepansky, Chicago and London: University of Chicago Press.

Kotsch, W. (2000) 'Jung's mediatory science as a psychology beyond objectivism', *Journal of Analytical Psychology*, 45(2): 217–44.

Lakoff, G. (1987) *Women, Fire and Dangerous Things: What Categories Reveal about the Mind*, Chicago: University of Chicago Press.

Lazarus, R. (1991) *Emotion and Adaptation*, New York and Oxford: Oxford University Press.

LeDoux, J. (1998) *The Emotional Brain*, London: Weidenfeld & Nicolson.

Lemaire, A. (1977) *Jacques Lacan*, London: Routledge & Kegan Paul.

Leslie, A. (1988) 'The necessity of illusion: perception and thought in infancy', in L. Weiskrantz (ed.) *Thought without Language*, Oxford: Clarendon.

Levi, P. (1977) *The Noise Made by Poems*, London: Anvil Press Poetry.

Lichtenberg, J. (1981) 'Implications for psychoanalytic theory of research on the neonate', *International Review of Psychoanalysis*, 8(1): 35–54.

Lieberman, A. (1999) 'Negative maternal attributions: effects on toddlers' sense of self', *Psychoanalytic Inquiry*, 19(5): 737–54.

Lindsay, D.A. (1906) *Plato: The Republic*, London: J.M. Dent.

Locke, J. (1997[1689]) *An Essay Concerning Human Understanding*, edited by R. Woolhouse, London: Penguin.

Lorenz, K. (1979) *The Year of the Greylag Goose*, London: Eyre Methuen.

McDowell, M. (2001) 'Principles of organization: a dynamic-systems view of the archetype-as-such', *Journal of Analytical Psychology*, 46(4): 637–54.

MacLean, P.D. (1949) 'Psychosomatic disease and the "visceral brain": recent developments bearing on the Papez theory of emotion', *Psychosomatic Medicine*, 2: 338–53.

McLynn, F. (1996) *Carl Gustav Jung*, London: Bantam.

Mahler, M. (1975) *The Psychological Birth of the Human Infant: Symbiosis and Individuation*, London: Maresfield Library/Karnac.

Main, M. and Cassidy, J. (in press) 'Adult attachment rating and classification systems', in M. Main (ed.) *A Typology of Human Attachment Organization Assessed in Discourse, Drawings and Interviews*, New York: Cambridge University Press.

Main, M. and Goldwyn, S. (1995) 'Interview-based adult attachment classification: related to infant–mother and infant–father attachment', *Developmental Psychology*, 19: 227–39.

Mandler, G. (1975) *Mind and Body: Psychology of Emotion and Stress*, New York and London: W.W. Norton.

Mandler, J. (1988) 'How to build a baby: on the development of an accessible representational system', *Cognitive Development*, 3: 113–36.

—— (1992) 'How to build a baby II: conceptual primitives', *Psychological Review*, 99(4): 587–604.

Marcel, A.J. (1983) 'Conscious and unconscious perception: an approach to the relations between phenomenal experience and perceptual processes', *Cognitive Psychology*, 15: 238–300.

—— (1988) 'Phenomenal experience and functionalism', in A.J. Marcel and E. Bisiach (eds) *Consciousness in Contemporary Science*, Oxford: Clarendon Press.

Marvin, R., Cooper, G., Hoffman, K. and Powell, B. (2002) 'The Circle of Security project: attachment-based intervention with caregiver–preschool child dyads', *Attachment and Human Development*, 4(1): 107–24.

Marx, K. (1995[1887]) *Capital*, Oxford: Oxford University Press, originally published (1887) F. Engels (ed.), trans. S. Moore and E. Aveling, London: Swan Sonnenschein.

Meltzer, D. (1973) *Sexual States of Mind*, Perthshire: Clunie Press.

Mitchell, S. (2002) 'Response to the JAP's questionnaire', *Journal of Analytical Psychology*, 47(1): 83–90.

Morgan, C. (1884) 'Instinct', *Nature*, 29: 370–4.

Nagy, M. (1991) *Philosophical Issues in the Psychology of C.G. Jung*, New York: State University of New York Press.

Nelson, K. (1999) 'Event representation, narrative development and internal working models', *Attachment and Human Development*, 1(3): 239–52.

Nesse, R.M. and Lloyd, A.T. (1992) 'The evolution of psychodynamic mechanisms', in J.H. Barkow, L. Cosmides and J. Tooby (eds) *The Adapted Mind: Evolutionary Psychology and the Generation of Culture*, New York and Oxford: Oxford University Press.

Noll, R. (1994) *The Jung Cult: Origins of a Charismatic Movement*, Princeton, NJ: Princeton University Press.

Panksepp, J. (1998) *Affective Neuroscience*, New York: Oxford University Press.

Papadopoulos, R. (1984) 'Jung and the concept of the Other', in R. Papadopoulos and G. Saayman (eds) *Jung in Modern Perspective*, London: Wildwood House.

Patrick, M., Hobson, R.P., Castle, D., Howard, R. and Maughan, B. (1994) 'Personality disorder and the mental representation of early social experience', *Developmental Psychology*, 6: 375–88.

Perlow, M. (1995) *Understanding Mental Objects*, London and New York: Routledge.

Perner, J., Leekam, S.R. and Wimmer, H. (1987) 'Three-year olds' difficulty with false belief: the case for a conceptual deficit', *British Journal of Developmental Psychology*, 5: 125–37.

Perry, C. (1997) 'Transference and countertransference', in P. Young-Eisendrath and T. Dawson (eds) *The Cambridge Companion to Jung*, Cambridge: Cambridge University Press.

Perry, P.D. (1999) 'The memories of states: how the brain stores and retrieves traumatic experience', in J.M. Goodwin and R. Attias (eds) *Splintered Reflections: Images of the Body in Trauma*, New York: Basic Books.

Pietikainen, P. (1998) 'Archetypes as symbolic forms', *Journal of Analytical Psychology*, 43(3): 325–449.

Pinker, S. (1994a) *The Language Instinct: The New Science of Language and Mind*, London: Allen Lane/The Penguin Press.

—— (1994b) 'On language', *Journal of Cognitive Neuroscience*, 6(1): 92–7.

—— (1997) *How the Mind Works*, London: Allen Lane/The Penguin Press.

Piontelli, A. (1992) *From Fetus to Child: An Observational and Psychoanalytic Study*, London and New York: Tavistock/Routledge.

Rauhala, L. (1984) 'The basic views of Jung in the light of hermeneutic metascience', in R. Papadopoulos and G. Saayman (eds) *Jung in Modern Perspective*, London: Wildwood House.

Rayner, E. (1992) 'John Bowlby's contribution, a brief survey', *Bulletin of the British Psychoanalytic Society*, 20(3).

Renik, O. (2000) 'Subjectivity and unconsciousness', *Journal of Analytical Psychology*, 45(1): 3–20.

Romanes, G. (1904[1882]) *Animal Intelligence*, London: Kegan Paul, Trench, Trubner & Co.

Rosenfeld, H. (1987) *Impasse and Interpretation: Therapeutic and Antitherapeutic Factors in the Psychoanalytic Treatment of Psychotic, Borderline, and Neurotic Patients*, London and New York: Tavistock.

Rycroft, C. (1979) *The Innocence of Dreams*, London: Hogarth Press.

Samuels, A. (1985) *Jung and the Post-Jungians*, London: Routledge & Kegan Paul.

Sander, L.W. (2002) 'Thinking differently: principles of process in living systems and the specificity of being known', *Psychoanalytic Dialogues*, 12(1): 11–42.

Sandler, J. and Dreher, A-U. (1996) *What do Psychoanalysts Want? The Problem of Aims in Psychoanalytic Psychotherapy*, London and New York: Routledge.

Sandler, J. and Joffe, W.G. (1967) 'The tendency to persistence in psychological function and development, with special reference to fixation and regression', *Bulletin Menninger Clinic*, 31: 257–71.

Sandner, D.F. and Beebe, J. (1984) 'Psychopathology and analysis', in M. Stein (ed.) *Jungian Analysis*, Boulder, CO and London: Shambhala.

Satinover, J. (1985) *At the Mercy of Another: Abandonment and Restitution in Psychosis and Psychotic Character*, Wilmette, IL: Chiron.

Saunders, P. and Skar, P. (2001) 'Archetypes, complexes and self-organization', *Journal of Analytical Psychology*, 46(2): 255–413.

Schacter, D. (1996) *Searching for Memory: The Brain, the Mind and the Past*, New York: Basic Books.

Schafer, R. (1999) 'Some reflections on the concept of enactment', in P. Fonagy, A. Cooper and R. Wallerstein (eds) *Psychoanalysis on the Move: The Work of Joseph Sandler*, New York and London: Routledge.

Schopenhauer, A. (1958) *World as Will and Representation*, vol. 1, trans. E.F.J. Payne, Dover: Falcon Wings Press.

Schore, A. (1994) *Affect Regulation and the Origins of the Self: The Neurobiology of Emotional Development*, Hillsdale, NJ: Lawrence Erlbaum.

—— (2000a) 'Attachment and the regulation of the right brain', *Attachment and Human Development*, 2(1): 23–7.

—— (2000b) 'Minds in the making: attachment, the self-organizing brain and developmentally-orientated psychoanalytic psychotherapy', *British Journal of Psychotherapy*, 17(3): 299–327.

Sebel, P. (1995) 'Memory during anaesthesia: gone but not forgotten', *Anaesthesia and Analgesia*, 81(4): 668.

Segal, H. (1986[1981]) *The Work of Hannah Segal: A Kleinian Approach to Clinical Practice*, London: Free Association, original publisher Jason Aronson.

Skinner, B.F. (1953) *Science and Human Behaviour*, London: Macmillan.

Sparks, J. (1982) *The Discovery of Animal Behaviour*, London: Collins.

Spillius, E.B. (1994) 'Developments in Kleinian thought: overview and personal view', *Psychoanalytic Inquiry*, 14: 324–64.

Sroufe, L.A. and Waters, E. (1977) 'Attachment as an organizational construct', *Child Development*, 48: 1184–99.

Steele, H., Steele, M. and Fonagy, P. (1996) 'Associations among attachment classifications of mothers, fathers and their infants', *Child Development*, 67: 541–55.

Stephens, B. (2001) 'The Martin Buber–Carl Jung disputation: protecting the sacred in the battle for the boundaries of analytical psychology', *Journal of Analytical Psychology*, 46(3): 455–92.

Stern, D. (1985) *The Interpersonal World of the Infant: A View from Psychoanalysis and Developmental Psychology*, New York: Basic Books.

—— (1994) 'One way to build a clinically relevant baby', *Infant Mental Health Journal*, 15: 36–54.

Stern, D., Bruschweiler-Stern, N., Harrison, A.M., Lyons-Ruth, K., Morgan, A.C., Nahum, J.P., Sander, L. and Tronick, E.Z. (1998) 'The process of therapeutic change involving implicit knowledge: some implications of developmental observations for adult psychotherapy', *Infant Mental Health Journal*, 19: 300–8.

Stevens, A. (1982) *Archetype: A Natural History of the Self*, London: Routledge and Kegan Paul.

—— (1990) *On Jung*, London and New York: Routledge.

—— (2000) 'Jungian analysis and evolutionary psychotherapy: an integrative approach', in P. Gilbert and K.B. Bailey (eds) *Genes on the Couch: Explorations in Evolutionary Psychology*, Hove: Brunner-Routledge.

—— (2002) *Archetype Revisited: An Updated Natural History of the Self*, London: Brunner-Routledge.

Storr, A. (1973) *Jung*, London: Fontana/Collins.

—— (1983) *The Essential Jung. Selected Writings*, Princeton, NJ: Princeton University Press.

Tronick, E.Z. (2002) 'A model of infant mood states and Sanderian affective waves', *Psychoanalytic Dialogues*, 12(1): 73–99.

Van der Kolk, B.A. and Fisler, R. (1995) 'Dissociation and the fragmentary nature of traumatic memories: overview and exploratory study', *Journal of Traumatic Stress*, 8(4): 505–25.

Vaughan, S., Spitzer, R., Davies, M. and Roose, S. (1997) 'The definition and assessment of analytic process: can analysts agree?', *International Journal of Psychoanalysis*, 78(5): 959–74.

Vidal, F. (2001) 'Sabina Spielrein, Jean Piaget: going their own ways', *Journal of Analytical Psychology*, 46(1): 139–54.

Von Franz, M. (1975) *C.G. Jung: His Myth in Our Time*, London: Hodder & Stoughton.

Weinshel, E.M. (1990) 'How wide is the widening scope of psychoanalysis and how solid is its structural model? Some concerns and observations', *Journal of the American Psychoanalytic Association*, 38: 272–96.

Weiskrantz, L. (1986) *Blindsight: A Case Study and Implications*, Oxford Psychology Series 12, Oxford: Oxford University Press.

Wheeley, S. (1992) 'Looks that kill the capacity for thought', *Journal of Analytical Psychology*, 37(2): 187–210.

Whittle, P. (1999) 'Experimental psychology and psychoanalysis: what we can learn from a century of misunderstanding', *Neuropsychoanalysis*, 1(2): 233–45.

Wilkinson, M. (2003) 'Undoing trauma. Contemporary neuroscience: a Jungian clinical perspective', *Journal of Analytical Psychology*.

Williams, M. (1963) 'The indivisibility of the personal and collective unconscious', in *Analytical Psychology: A Modern Science*, London: Library of Analytical Psychology/William Heinemann.

Winnicott, D.W. (1971[1967]) 'Mirror role of the mother and family in child development', in *Playing and Reality*, London: Tavistock, originally published in P. Lomas (ed.) *The Predicament of the Family: A Psychoanalytical Symposium*, London: Hogarth Press.

—— (1971) *Playing and Reality*, London: Tavistock.

—— (1975[1951]) 'Transitional objects and transitional phenomena', in *Through Paediatrics to Psycho-Analysis*, London: Hogarth Press.

Index